MANAGEMENT OF VERTIGO
Made Easy®

MANAGEMENT OF VERTIGO
Made Easy®

Santosh Kumar Swain
MS (ENT) DNB (ENT) MNAMS Fellowship in Neuro-otology

Associate Professor
Department of Otorhinolaryngology
Institute of Medical Sciences and SUM Hospital
Siksha O Anusandhan University
Bhubaneswar, Odisha, India

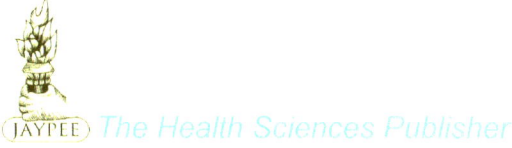

New Delhi | London | Philadelphia | Panama

Jaypee Brothers Medical Publishers (P) Ltd.

Headquarters

Jaypee Brothers Medical Publishers (P) Ltd.
4838/24, Ansari Road, Daryaganj
New Delhi 110 002, India
Phone: +91-11-43574357
Fax: +91-11-43574314
E-mail: jaypee@jaypeebrothers.com

Overseas Offices

J.P. Medical Ltd.
83, Victoria Street, London
SW1H 0HW (UK)
Phone: +44 20 3170 8910
Fax: +44 (0)20 3008 6180
E-mail: info@jpmedpub.com

Jaypee-Highlights Medical Publishers Inc.
City of Knowledge, Bld. 237, Clayton
Panama City, Panama
Phone: +1 507-301-0496
Fax: +1 507-301-0499
E-mail: cservice@jphmedical.com

Jaypee Medical Inc.
325 Chestnut Street
Suite 412, Philadelphia, PA 19106, USA
Phone: +1 267-519-9789
E-mail: jpmed.us@gmail.com

Jaypee Brothers Medical Publishers (P) Ltd.
17/1-B, Babar Road, Block-B, Shaymali
Mohammadpur, Dhaka-1207
Bangladesh
Mobile: +08801912003485
E-mail: jaypeedhaka@gmail.com

Jaypee Brothers Medical Publishers (P) Ltd.
Bhotahity, Kathmandu, Nepal
Phone: +977-9741283608
E-mail: kathmandu@jaypeebrothers.com

Website: www.jaypeebrothers.com
Website: www.jaypeedigital.com

© 2016, Jaypee Brothers Medical Publishers

The views and opinions expressed in this book are solely those of the original contributor(s)/author(s) and do not necessarily represent those of editor(s) of the book.

All rights reserved. No part of this publication may be reproduced, stored or transmitted in any form or by any means, electronic, mechanical, photocopying, recording or otherwise, without the prior permission in writing of the publishers.

All brand names and product names used in this book are trade names, service marks, trademarks or registered trademarks of their respective owners. The publisher is not associated with any product or vendor mentioned in this book.

Medical knowledge and practice change constantly. This book is designed to provide accurate, authoritative information about the subject matter in question. However, readers are advised to check the most current information available on procedures included and check information from the manufacturer of each product to be administered, to verify the recommended dose, formula, method and duration of administration, adverse effects and contraindications. It is the responsibility of the practitioner to take all appropriate safety precautions. Neither the publisher nor the author(s)/editor(s) assume any liability for any injury and/or damage to persons or property arising from or related to use of material in this book.

This book is sold on the understanding that the publisher is not engaged in providing professional medical services. If such advice or services are required, the services of a competent medical professional should be sought.

Every effort has been made where necessary to contact holders of copyright to obtain permission to reproduce copyright material. If any have been inadvertently overlooked, the publisher will be pleased to make the necessary arrangements at the first opportunity.

Inquiries for bulk sales may be solicited at: jaypee@jaypeebrothers.com

Management of Vertigo Made Easy®

First Edition: **2016**
ISBN: 978-93-5250-029-1

Dedicated to

My parents who gave me life and a value
My teachers who gave me knowledge and a profession, and
My patients who gave me appreciation and encouragement.

Preface

For the most medical practitioners, a heart-sinking moment is inevitable when confronted by a patient presenting with vertigo. The diagnosis and management of vertigo have always been an enigma because of the complexity of the balance system and inherent compensatory mechanisms as well as redundancy of functions render the system immune to most diagnostic tests. *Management of Vertigo Made Easy*® is written for everybody who wants to learn vertigo and treat dizzy patients. Medical students, interns, residents, primary care physicians, and consultants can use this book for proper management of vertigo patients. The most important point in managing vertigo patient is always to take good history. This is followed by appropriate examinations and investigations. Basic concepts in assessing, diagnosing and managing common peripheral vestibular disorders are briefly described, and special emphasis is given on how to rule out central vertigo. The book is a reader's delight and is sure to spark an interest in managing vertigo patients.

Santosh Kumar Swain

Acknowledgments

I am deeply indebted to my teacher and mentor Professors (Drs) Abhoy Kar, GC Sahoo, SN Panda, RN Samal, S Behera, RK Pattnaik, and KC Mallick, Souvagini Acharya, and Satyajit Mishra for their great moral support in writing this book.

I sincerely thank President Manoj Ranjan Nayak and Management Member Er GB Kar, Siksha 'O' Anusandhan University, Bhubaneswar, Odisha, for their great support behind this work.

I heartily thank Shri Jitendar P Vij (Group Chairman), Mr Ankit Vij (Group President) and Mr Tarun Duneja (Director-Publishing) of M/s Jaypee Brothers Medical Publishers (P) Ltd, New Delhi, India, for strong belief in the book for benefiting the medical fraternity.

I can never forget people, who came in my professional training to teach, appreciate and encourage my hard work, Professors Anand Job, Rita Ruby Albert, Achma Balraj, Rupa Vedanta, Christian Medical College, Vellore, Tamil Nadu, India.

I am very much thankful to Mahesh Ch Sahu, Somadatta Das of Central Research Laboratory, and Manoj Mishra and Susanta Kumar Khuntia of Central Library, for their help in editing the manuscript.

My patients are the another source of inspiration for attempting to write vertigo in simple and lucid manner.

Last but not least, I am grateful to my parents, wife (Swagatika) and son (Ishan), without their encouragement and cooperation, the book could never have been written.

Contents

1. **Introduction**   1
   Definition of Vertigo *2*
   Classification *2*
   Vertigo Pearls *3*
   Quality of Life in Vertigo Patient *4*

2. **Physiology of Vertigo**   5
   Functional Anatomy *5*
   Basic Physiology of Balance Disorder *8*

3. **Causes of Vertigo**   11
   Peripheral Causes *11*
   Central Causes *13*
   Peripheral Vestibular Disorders *13*
   Labyrinthine Vertigo *16*
   Central Vestibular Disorders *17*
   Basics of Peripheral Vertigo *21*
   Epidemiology of Peripheral Vertigo *21*
   Basics of Central Vertigo *21*
   Epidemiology of Central Vertigo *21*
   Physiological Vertigo *22*
   Drugs Causing Dizziness *23*
   Ototoxicity and Dizziness *23*
   Old Age and Dizziness *24*

Dizziness in Children *24*
Dizziness in Pregnancy *25*
Post-Traumatic Vertigo *25*

4. Diagnosis of Vertigo from History — 28

Things about Dizzy Spells *28*
Assess the Problem *29*
History Tells Diagnosis *29*
Vertigo Diagnosis *35*

5. Clinical Tests for Vertigo — 37

Routine Examinations for Vertigo Patients *37*
Special Vestibular Tests *50*
Oculomotor Tests *52*
Cerebellar Tests *53*
Tests for Utricular/Otolithic Dysfunction *53*

6. Investigations for Vertigo — 55

Hematological Tests *55*
Audiological Test *55*
Radiological Tests *55*
Glycerol Test *56*
Special Vestibular Investigations *57*
Conditions Requiring Urgent Neuroimaging (CT/MRI) *61*

7. Treatment of Vertigo — 62

Objective of Treatment *62*
Principles of Management of Vertigo *62*

Rotatory Vertigo 66
Episodic for Hours 67
Prolonged Rotatory 68
Unsteadiness 69
Medications in Central Vertigo 75
Particle Repositioning and Exercises for BPPV 76

8. **Vestibular Rehabilitation Exercises** **85**
Mechanisms 85
Cawthrone-Cooksey Exercises 86
Eye Exercises 86
Head and Neck Exercises 86

9. **Important Clinical Conditions of Vertigo** **96**
Ménière's Disease 96
Benign Paroxysmal Positional Vertigo 99
Vestibular Neuronitis 99
Perilymph Fistula 100
Superior Semicircular Canal Dehiscence 101
Labyrinthitis 102
Acoustic Neuroma 102
Bilateral Vestibulopathy 103
Autoimmune Labyrinthitis 104
Central Causes of Vertigo 104
Motion Sickness 107

10. **Approach to Vertigo by General Practitioner** **110**
Diagnosis of Otologic Vertigo 111
Conditions Requiring Urgent
Referral to Balance Specialist 111

Simplified Approach to Get a Diagnosis *111*
   Guiding for Evaluation of Dizzy Patients *115*

11. Interesting Case Series   **119**

   Case 1: Vestibular Neuronitis *119*

   Case 2: Ménière's Disease *120*

   Case 3: Benign Paroxysmal Positional Vertigo *122*

   Case 4: Ménière's Disease *123*

   Case 5: Migraine-related Vertigo *123*

   Case 6: Perilymph Fistula *126*

   Case 7 *127*

   Case 8 *128*

   Case 9 *129*

   Case 10 *130*

12. Vertigo Clinic Evaluation Format   **131**

   History *131*

   Examinations *134*

   Investigations *136*

   Management *136*

Points to Remember   *137*

Bibliography   *149*

Index   *151*

CHAPTER 1

Introduction

Vertigo and dizziness are extremely common problem, but are often misdiagnosed. The problem occurs because patients use the term very loosely to describe a broad variety of unpleasant and unfamiliar sensations, including spinning, faintness, unsteadiness and numbness or lightheadedness. The only common feature is a feeling of uncertainty of position or motion.

Vertigo is a feeling in which the external world seems to revolve around the individual or in which the individual seems to revolve in space. Vertigo is not a disease but is a symptom. Vertigo is a very distressing symptom not only for patients but also for the treating doctors. It is a challenging problem for diagnosis and treatment. It is prevalent amongst 10% of the patients visited by an ENT specialist. It is 5% of patients visiting the general practitioner are suffering from the vertigo. For treatment of vertigo, most of the patients run among neurologists, ophthalmologists, otolaryngologists, orthopedicians and general physicians and finally frustrated and seek advice from psychiatrists. This book is a honest trial for making simplification of vertigo approach and give justice to dizzy patient.

The basic aim of this book is to answer:
- Does the subject really have a balance disorder?
- If so, whether it is a central or peripheral disorder?
- What is the probable etiology?
- What is the best possible treatment?

DEFINITION OF VERTIGO

- Vertigo is defined as a subjective sense of imbalance.
- Vertigo is defined by Cawthorne (1957) as a *Hallucination of movement and can be applied to any movement provided that it does not exist outside the sense of sufferer.*
- True vertigo is a sense of rotation of one's body or head (subjective), or of the environment (objective), or sense of falling.
- Vertigo may be defined as a hallucination of movement, that is the patients feel that they or their environments are moving.
- Vertigo could be defined as a false sense of orientation of the patient with respect to his environment. The patient feels that he is moving or that the surroundings are moving.
- A balance disorder/vertigo is a medical condition that causes an individual to feel unsteady when standing or walking and may be accompanied by feelings of giddiness or woozings or having a sensation of movement, spinning or floating.

Vertigo is often thought to be synonymous with dizziness. Vertigo is a sensation of disorientation in space along with a sensation of motion. Dizziness is an imbalance usually associated with cardiovascular, neurosensory and psychiatric conditions and few medications.

Visual, proprioception and vestibular systems coordinate with the central nervous system (CNS) to maintain equilibrium and provide a sense of spatial orientation. Any disease that disrupts this system leads to vertigo and disequilibrium.

CLASSIFICATION

All dizzy patients can be divided into those who are spinning and those who have a sense of unsteadiness.

Sensation of rotation is subdivided further into those in whom it lasts for hours. We almost never get a patient coming and complaining of two minutes of dizziness. It is usually significantly less or significantly longer. And of course the prolonged can last for weeks or months or even forever.

- *Sensation of rotation:*
  - Episodic—seconds/hours
  - Prolonged—weeks.
- *Sensation of unsteadiness:*
  - Episodic—seconds/hours to days
  - Prolonged—weeks to months or forever.

The sensation of rotation most commonly arises from a problem within the labyrinth whereas the sensation of unsteadiness is more a problem within the whole system rather than especially localized to the labyrinth.

Remember during Managing the Vertigo Patients

- Advice patient not to be panic.
- Underlying causes of the most of vertigo are simple.
- Most of them do not require admission in intensive care.
- Do not advice costly investigations such as computed tomography (CT), magnetic resonance imaging (MRI), etc. until really indicated.
- Learn the art of the history taking for diagnosis of vertigo.
- Think about common causes first.

VERTIGO PEARLS

- *Vertigo:* It is a symptom, not disease.
- History gives the diagnosis in 90% cases.
- Majority of the cases are peripheral.
- Have low threshold for suspecting TIA/stroke.
- Do not be reassured with a normal CT/MRI.
- Use vestibular suppressants judiciously and only for few days, if there is disabling rotatory vertigo. Never prescribe vestibular suppressants for imbalance/ataxia as it worsens the situation.

- *Judicious use of newer technology:* Videonystagmography (VNG), MRI and special chairs.

Prevalence of Vertigo in Community

- Vertigo is being reported to occur in 25% of middle-aged population and about 40% in elderly.
- By the age of 75 years, dizziness is the most common cause for seeking medical advice.
- It is the ninth most common cause for primary care physician visits.
- As per *American Institute of Health Statistics* data, 50% of all accidental death from fall above 65 years is due to balance disorder.

QUALITY OF LIFE IN VERTIGO PATIENT

Quality of life is hampered in vertigo patients. Factors that affect quality of life in patients with vertigo are:
- Agoraphobia.
- Social impairment.
- Depression.
- Anxiety neurosis.
- Drug side effects.
- 3Fs syndrome (Fear of frequent falling).

There is always a need to develop a systematic, efficient and formal assessment strategy for the diagnosis of the symptom complex of dizziness or vertigo and disequilibrium is paramount in order to provide appropriate management and rehabilitation.

CHAPTER 2

Physiology of Vertigo

The ability to maintain balance is essential to nearly all activities associated with daily livings. Maintenance of balance is a dynamic process involving the vestibular system, the visual system, the proprioceptive system and the central nervous system. Considering the complexity of these mechanisms of postural control, it is indeed amazing that the sense of maintaining balance does not surface to our awareness in daily life. We become aware of posture and balance only when there is a malfunction of any or all the components involved.

FUNCTIONAL ANATOMY

Vestibular system has two components—peripheral and central. Central vestibular system consists of vestibular nuclei, connections of vestibular nuclei to cerebellum, spinal cord and extraocular motor nuclei. Peripheral vestibular system consists of labyrinth. The labyrinth (**Figs 2.1A and B**) consists of vestibule, semicircular canals and vestibular nerves. Utricle and saccule constitutes the vestibule. The labyrinth has bony and membranous part. The membranous labyrinth contains hair cells that sense the motion of head. The hair cells are located in the ampulla of the three semicircular canals and in the macula of the utricle and saccule.

The hair cells of the semicircular canals are stimulated only when there is an angular acceleration. The hair cells of the utricle are stimulated, when the head moves forward or backward, and the hair cells of the saccule are stimulated when the head

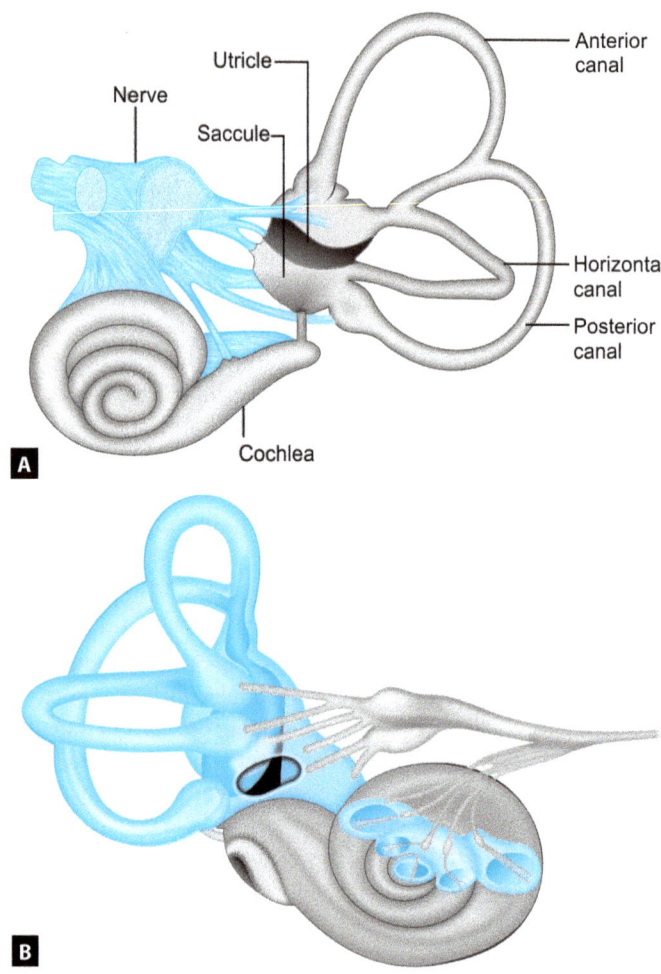

Figs 2.1A and B Inner ear and its parts

Physiology of Vertigo

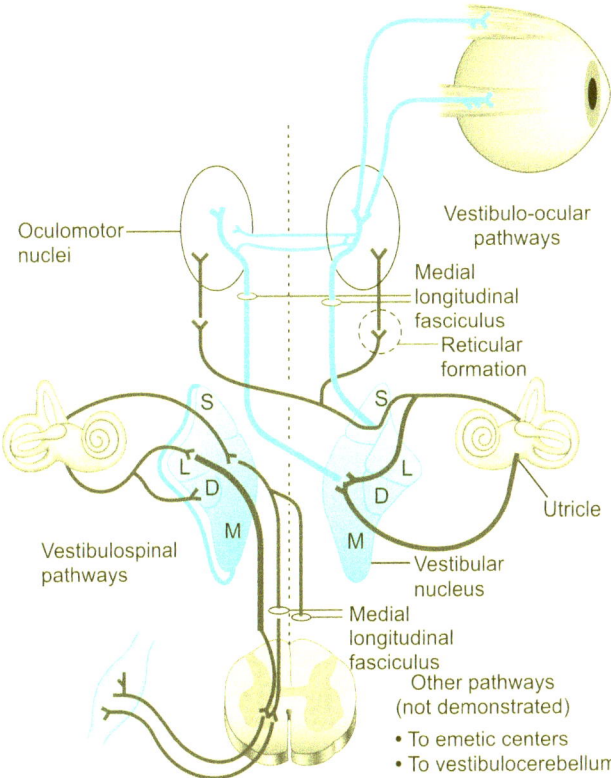

Fig. 2.2 Vestibular nuclei and their connections (Vestibular pathway)

moves sideways. The utricle and saccule sense gravitational orientation and linear acceleration.

The sensory impulses from the labyrinth travel through the vestibular nerve to reach the Scarpa's ganglion. From Scarpa's ganglion, the impulses are relayed to vestibular nuclei. There are four vestibular nuclei (**Fig. 2.2**): Superior (Bechterew's nucleus), inferior (spinal nucleus), medial (Schwalbe's nucleus) and lateral (nucleus of Deiters). Superior nucleus is situated at pons. Inferior nucleus is at lower medulla, medial nucleus is at floor of fourth ventricle (medulla) and lateral nucleus is at upper medulla. The superior vestibular nuclei transmit impulses to medial longitudinal fasciculus (MLF), and hence to the 3rd, 4th and 6th cranial nerve nuclei. From lateral vestibular nuclei, impulses are transmitted to brainstem from where it reaches spinal cords to control muscles of extremities. Medial and inferior vestibular nuclei relay impulses to medial longitudinal fasciculus and then to reticular formation and 11th cranial nerve nucleus respectively.

CLINICAL TIPS

Labyrinth contains two main sensory end organs which help in maintaining balance, i.e. utricle and semicircular canals. Utricle by gravitational pull of its chalk particles give information about position of head in space. Semicircular canals give information about the change of position of head in space.

BASIC PHYSIOLOGY OF BALANCE DISORDER

The balance system is a complex multiorgan and multisystem mechanism. The central nervous system, the peripheral nervous system, the musculoskeletal system, the visual system and of course, the vestibular system, all work in tandem to maintain the body's balance (**Fig. 2.3**).

The information about the spatial orientation (i.e. position of the body in relation to the ground and surroundings) is provided to the central nervous system from three sources the vestibular labyrinths of the two sides, the two eyes and the sensory receptors called proprioceptors in the muscles of the limbs (mainly the lower limbs)—the neck and trunk. The central nervous system integrates the information from these three sources and in response to it, generates a motor reaction. Motor reaction or response means a contraction of the requisite muscles in the body so that the subject

Physiology of Vertigo

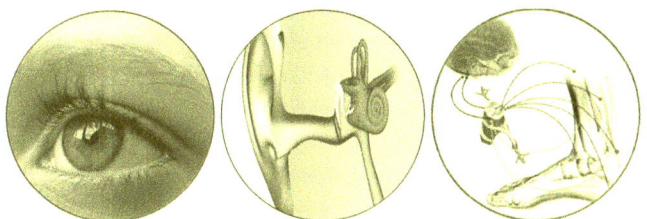

Fig. 2.3 Components responsible for maintaining balance

can effectively maintain his posture without falling, despite sudden changes in the subject's position or in his environment. The accuracy of timing, preciseness and perfect coordination of the muscular contraction of the extraocular and skeletal muscles is maintained by the cerebellum.

The vestibular labyrinth has a basic resting activity which discharges impulses at a steady rate even in the absence of an external stimulus and is responsible for maintaining muscle tone. The resting activity from each labyrinth tends to deviate the eyes and the body to the opposite sides being normally equal, a state of balance is maintained. For example, the resting activity of the right vestibular labyrinth tries to move the eyes to the left, while that of the left vestibular labyrinth tries to move them to right. The two forces or actions being equal, balance each other and hence no eye movement occurs. The same is true for the muscles of the neck and the trunk. Physiological or pathological stimuli that upset this balance between the two sides will produce a state of disequilibrium, leading to nystagmus and body deviation.

Two key pathways from the vestibular apparatus are involved in the maintenance of gaze and posture, i.e. the vestibulo-ocular reflex (VOR) and the vestibulospinal reflex (VSR). Vestibular pathways and their cardinal features are given in **Table 2.1**.

Management of Vertigo Made Easy

Table 2.1 Vestibular pathways and their cardinal features	
Pathways	Cardinal features
Vestibulo-ocular reflex (VOR)	Nystagmus
Vestibulospinal tracts (VSTs)	Falling to side
Vestibulocerebellar tracts (VCTs)	Ataxia, past pointing
Emetic pathways	Nausea, vomiting
Parietotemporal cortex	Vertigo

Any disturbance in labyrinth or vision or proprioception leads to balance disorder.

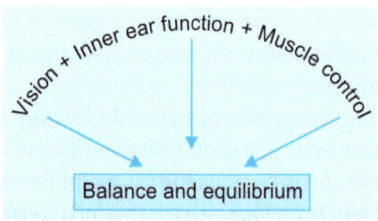

Vertigo is usually considered as a difficult problem to manage as a vast variety of causes may be involved in causing imbalance such as:
- Otological problems.
- Visual problems.
- Locomotive system disturbances (Proprioceptive system).
- Central nervous system.
- Cardiovascular system.

CHAPTER 3

Causes of Vertigo

Disorders of the vestibular system can be divided into: (A) Peripheral vestibular origin, and (B) Central origin.

Peripheral causes: It involves vestibular end organs and their first order neurons (vestibular nerve). The cause lies in the inner ear or the 8th nerve.

Central causes: It involves the central nervous system after the entrance of vestibular nerve in the brainstem and involves vestibule-ocular, vestibule-spinal and other central nervous system pathways.

Common causes of dizziness are provided in **Box 3.1**.

PERIPHERAL CAUSES

Lesions of end organs and vestibular nerve
- Ménière's disease.
- Benign paroxysmal positional vertigo (BPPV).
- Vestibular neuronitis.
- Labyrinthitis.
- Perilymph fistula.
- Vestibulotoxic drugs.
- Syphilis.
- Acoustic neuroma.

Box 3.1 Common causes of dizziness

Peripheral vestibular disorders
- Benign paroxysmal positional vertigo
- Ménière's disease
- Vestibular neuritis
- Labyrinthitis
- Perilymph fistula
- Bilateral vestibulopathy

Central disorders
- Cervical vertigo
- Traumatic head injury
- Migraine
- Multiple sclerosis
- Anterior or posterior inferior cerebellar stroke
- Transient ischemic attacks
- Post-traumatic anxiety symptoms
- Vestibular ocular dysfunction

Psychiatric disorders
- Panic disorders
- Agoraphobia
- Hyperventilation syndrome

Other causes
- Presyncope
- Low blood pressure
- Arrhythmias
- Vertebral artery trauma
- Alternobaric vertigo
- Diabetes mellitus
- Thyroid dysfunction
- Human immune deficiency virus
- Syphilitic labyrinthitis
- Epstein-Barr virus
- Brainstem hemorrhage
- Friedreich's ataxia
- Recent diplopia
- Medications

Vertigo with Deafness

- Ménière's disease.
- Labyrinthitis.
- Acoustic neuroma.
- Labyrinthine trauma.
- Ototoxic vertigo.

Vertigo without Deafness

- Vestibular neuronitis.
- Benign paroxysmal positional vertigo.

CENTRAL CAUSES

- Lesions of brainstem and central connections.
- Posterior-inferior cerebellar artery syndrome.
- Vertebrobasilar insufficiency.
- Basilar migraine.
- Multiple sclerosis.
- Tumors of the brainstem and fourth ventricle.
- Epilepsy.
- Cervical vertigo.

PERIPHERAL VESTIBULAR DISORDERS

Ménière's Disease

- It is also called as endolymphatic hydrops (**Fig. 3.1**).
- It is characterized by vertigo, fluctuating sensorineural hearing loss, tinnitus and sense of fullness in the involved ear.
- Vertigo is of sudden onset.
- Vertigo lasts for a few minutes to 24 hours or so.

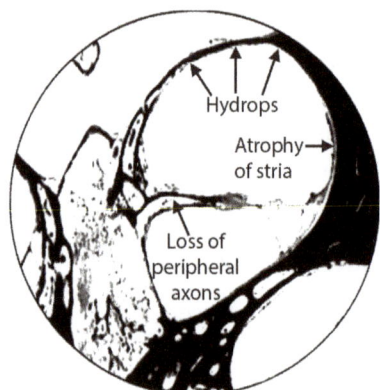

Fig. 3.1 Inner ear hydrops

Benign Paroxysmal Positional Vertigo (BPPV)

- It is characterized by the vertiginous episodes with the positional changes of head, usually in supine position with involved ear downwards.
- It is due to displacement of the otoconia, which tend to reach the posterior semicircular canal.
- The attack usually starts within 5 seconds and lasts for about one minute.
- There is rotatory nystagmus with quick component towards the involved ear.

Vestibular Neuronitis

- It is characterized by severe vertigo of sudden onset with no cochlear symptoms.
- Attack lasts for few days to 2 or 3 weeks.
- It is thought to occur due to a virus that attacks vestibular ganglion.

Labyrinthitis

- There is severe vertigo and sensorineural hearing loss.
- There is severe nausea and vomiting.
- Nystagmus is seen to the opposite side due to destruction of the affected labyrinth.
- Labyrinthitis is seen in unsafe type of chronic suppurative otitis media (CSOM).

Vestibulotoxic Drugs

- Aminoglycoside antibiotics, particularly streptomycin, gentamycin, kanamycin have shown to affect hair cells of the crista ampullaris and to some extent those of the maculae.
- Certain drugs which cause dizziness or unsteadiness are antihypertensive, labyrinthine sedatives, estrogen preparations, diuretics, antimicrobials (nalidixic acid, metronidazole) and antimalarials.

Head Injury

- Head injury may cause concussion of the labyrinth, completely disrupt the bony labyrinth or the 8th nerve or cause perilymph fistula.
- Severe acoustic trauma such as that caused by an explosion can also disrupt the vestibular end organ (otoliths) and result in vertigo.

Perilymph Fistula

- A perilymph fistula causes intermittent vertigo and fluctuating sensorineural hearing loss, sometimes with tinnitus and sense of fullness in the ear.
- In this condition, perilymph leaks into the middle ear through the oval or round window.

- It can follow as a complication of stapedectomy or ear surgery when stapes is accidently dislocated.
- It can also result from sudden pressure changes in the middle ear (e.g. barotraumas, diving, forceful Valsalva) or raised intracranial pressure (weightlifting or vigorous coughing).

Syphilis

- Syphilis of inner ear, both acquired and congenital causes dizziness in addition to sensorineural hearing loss.
- Late congenital syphilis usually manifests between 8 and 20 years, mimics Ménière's disease.
- Hennebert's sign, i.e. a positive fistula test in the presence of an intact tympanic membrane is present in congenital syphilis.
- Neurosyphilis (tertiary acquired) can cause central type of vestibular dysfunction.

Acoustic Neuroma

- It is a peripheral vestibular disorder as it arises from 8th cranial nerve within internal acoustic meatus.
- It causes only unsteadiness or vague sensation of motion.

LABYRINTHINE VERTIGO

Labyrinthine vertigo is classified into groups, i.e. due to
- Labyrinthine stimulation.
- Labyrinthine depression.

Both the types may be unilateral and bilateral.

Unilateral Labyrinthine Stimulation

Ear surgery: This can be a short period of postoperative dizziness due to stimulation of labyrinth for which all postoperative ontological cases should be assessed.

Caloric stimulation: This is usually seen in caloric test but may also occur in syringing the ear with water used at temperature above or below the normal body temperature, i.e. 37°C. So, proper care should be taken to assess the temperature of water used for syringing.

Benign paroxysmal positional vertigo (BPPV): It is the most common cause of vertigo encountered in day-to-day ENT practice.

Bilateral Labyrinthine Stimulation

It usually occurs in pseudophysiological condition in everyday life such as head spins, swings, travel sickness, etc.

Unilateral Incomplete Depression of Labyrinth

- Ménière's disease.
- Vestibular neuronitis.

Unilateral Complete Depression of Labyrinth

Trauma: This may due to head injury with transverse fracture of temporal bone or surgery with deliberate labyrinthectomy or accidental destruction of inner ear function in tympanoplasty or stapedotomy, etc.

Infections: Bacterial and viral labyrinthitis can cause sudden and complete destructive episode producing vertigo which behaves clinically in the same way.

Vascular: Vascular catastrophe affecting the inner ear can result in severe loss of labyrinthine function with/without loss of hearing. Various factors have to be taken into account such as atresia of vertebral artery, arteriosclerosis that may cause stenosis or occlusion of arteries and embolism occurring in both the arterial wall and heart.

Bilateral Complete Depression of Labyrinth

It may occur suddenly in vertebrobasilar disease and gradually with ototoxic drugs.

CENTRAL VESTIBULAR DISORDERS

Posterior Inferior Cerebellar Artery Syndrome (Wallenberg's Syndrome)

- There is thrombosis of the posteroinferior cerebellar artery cuts-off blood supply to lateral medullary area.
- There is violent vertigo along with diplopia, dysphagia, hoarseness of voice, Horner's syndrome, sensory loss on ipsilateral side of face and contralateral side of the body and ataxia.
- There may be horizontal or rotatory nystagmus to the side of the lesion.

Vertebrobasilar Insufficiency

- It is a common cause of central vertigo in patients above the age of 50 years.
- There is transient decrease in cerebral blood flow.
- Common cause is atherosclerosis.
- It may be precipitated by hypotension or neck movements, when cervical osteophytes press on the vertebral arteries during rotation and extension of the head.
- Vertigo is sudden in onset, lasts for several minutes and is associated with nausea and vomiting.
- Neurological symptoms such as visual disturbances, drop attacks, diplopia, hemianopia, dysphagia, hemiparesis due to ischemia of the other areas of the brain.
- Some may only complain intermittent attacks of dizziness or vertigo on lateral rotation and extension of the head.

Basilar Artery Migraine

- Basilar artery migraine produces occipital headache, visual disturbances, diplopia and severe vertigo which is abrupt and may last for 5–60 minutes.
- It is common in adolescent girls with strong menstrual relationship and positive family history.

Cerebellar Disease

- Acute cerebellar disease may cause severe vertigo, vomiting and ataxia simulating an acute peripheral labyrinthine disorder.
- Tumors in cerebellum are slow growing and produce classical features of cerebellar disease, i.e. incoordination, past-pointing, adiadochokinesia, rebound phenomenon and wide base gait.

Multiple Sclerosis

- It is a demyelinating disease affecting young adults.
- Vertigo and dizziness are common symptoms.
- Multiple neurological signs and symptoms like blurring or loss of vision, diplopia, dysarthria, paresthesia and ataxia.
- Spontaneous nystagmus may be seen.
- Acquired pendular nystagmus, dissociated nystagmus and vertical upbeat nystagmus are important features in diagnosis.

Tumors of Brainstem and Floor of Fourth Ventricle

- There are neurological signs and symptoms in addition to vertigo and dizziness.
- Positional vertigo and nystagmus may also be the presenting features.
- CT scan and MRI are useful in their diagnosis.

Temporal Lobe Epilepsy

- Vertigo may occur as an aura in temporal lobe epilepsy.
- History of seizure and /or unconsciousness following the aura may help in the diagnosis.
- Sometimes vertigo is the only symptom of epilepsy and that may create a difficult diagnostic problem. EEG may show abnormalities during the attack.

Cervical Vertigo

- It is a controversial diagnosis. At this point, it has not been established as a clear physiologically proven clinical entity.
- It may follow injuries of the neck.
- It is aggravated with movements of the neck to the side of the injury.
- X-ray shows cervical lordosis. On examination shows tenderness of the neck and spasm of the neck muscles and limited neck movement.
- Exact mechanism of vertigo is not known. It may be due to disturbed vertebrobasilar circulation, involvement of sympathetic vertebral plexus or alteration of tonic neck reflexes or inflammation of the deep cervical muscles or intervertebral ligaments.

Other Causes of Vertigo

- **Ocular vertigo:** Balance is maintained by the eyes, labyrinth and somatosensory system. A mismatch of information from any of these organs causes vertigo. Ocular vertigo may occur in case of sudden extraocular muscle paralysis or high errors of refraction.
- **Psychogenic vertigo**
  - This diagnosis is suspected when patients suffering from emotional tension and anxiety.

- Most of the times symptoms of neurosis, e.g. palpitation, breathlessness, fatigue, insomnia, profuse sweating and tremors are also present.
- Symptoms of vertigo are often vague in the form of floating or swimming sensation or light-headedness.
- There is no hearing loss or no nystagmus. Caloric test shows an exaggerated response.
• Anemia.
• Hypoglycemia.
• Orthostatic hypotension.

BASICS OF PERIPHERAL VERTIGO

False sensation of movement when no movement is actually occurring; results from peripheral causes such as inflammation, infection or other disorders of the ear or vestibular nerve.

EPIDEMIOLOGY OF PERIPHERAL VERTIGO

- It accounts for 54% of cases of dizziness reported in primary care.
- More than 90% of these patients are diagnosed with peripheral causes, such as BPPV.

BASICS OF CENTRAL VERTIGO

False sensation (hallucination) of movement originating from the central nervous system (CNS); results from hemorrhagic or ischemic injuries to the cerebellum, the vestibular nuclei and their connections within the brain stem, lesions of cranial nerve VII, intracranial neoplasms, infection, trauma and multiple sclerosis.

EPIDEMIOLOGY OF CENTRAL VERTIGO

- About 7–17% cases of vertigo are central in origin.
- Incidence of ischemic strokes primarily affecting the cerebellum is 1.5%.

- About 10% of patients with an isolated cerebellar infarction presents with only isolated vertigo and imbalance.
- Incidence of cerebrovascular disease (cerebellar infarction) is slightly higher in men than in women.
- Elderly patients have a higher incidence of central vertigo owing to increased incidence of cerebrovascular disease. The mean age of patients with cerebellar infarction is 60–80 years.

PHYSIOLOGICAL VERTIGO

- It includes motion sickness and height vertigo.
- It occurs when there is a mismatch between the vestibular, ocular and proprioceptive inputs due to an external stimulus (Unlike pathological vertigo which is due to a lesion in the vestibular pathway).

Motion Sickness

- It includes car sickness, sea sickness, flight sickness and space sickness.
- It is an acute disorder with symptoms appearing within minutes to hours of the stimulus and disappearing within hours after the stimuli.
- Reading in a moving or accelerating vehicle can cause this condition.
- Continuous exposure, as in sea travel leads to centrally mediated adaptation in about 3 days.
- Prevention by adaptation exercises with intermittent exposure to the stimulus.
- *Pharmacotherapy for motion sickness:* Meclizine, dimenhydrinate or scopolamine may benefit by inhibiting neuronal activity.
- Specific measures such as sitting in the front seat of the car, reducing accelerating movements may be of benefit.

Height Vertigo

Dizziness occurs when looking down from a great height or looking up a tall building or cliff.

DRUGS CAUSING DIZZINESS

- Aminoglycosides, cisplatin–damage vestibular hair cells → cause vertigo, disequilibrium.
- Antiepileptics (carbamazepine, phenytoin)–cause cerebellar toxicity → cause disequilibrium.
- Alcohol → CNS depression, cerebellar toxicity, changes in cupula specific gravity → cause disequilibrium and intoxication.
- Anticoagulants → cause hemorrhage into inner ear or brain → vertigo.
- Antihypertensives and diuretics → cause postural hypotension → faint like dizziness.
- Methotrexate → cause brainstem and cerebellar toxicity → cause disequilibrium.
- Parkinsonian drugs, e.g. bromocriptine, levodopa/carbidopa; muscle relaxants like baclofen → cause postural hypotension → leads to faint like sensation.
- Urologic drugs like sildenafil, oxybutynin → cause postural hypotension → faint like sensation.

OTOTOXICITY AND DIZZINESS

- Ototoxicity can cause vestibulotoxicity (damage to the vestibular apparatus) or cochleotoxicity (damage to the cochlea).
- Vestibulotoxicity causes vertigo while cochleotoxicity causes tinnitus and hearing loss.
- Topical ototoxicity occurs with antibiotic eardrops used for the treatment of chronic suppurative otitis media, where there is a perforated eardrum.

- Bilateral vestibular loss can occur with the use of systemic ototoxic agents, such as aminoglycoside antibiotics. This results in oscillopsia.

OLD AGE AND DIZZINESS

Dizziness is a common problem in the elderly and can lead to problems with balance, which in turns, results in falls with head injuries or long bone fractures. Different terms are used to describe dizziness among the elderly including multisensory dizziness, disequilibrium of aging or presbyastasis.

The cause is usually multifactorial and contributed by the following:
- From fifth decade onwards, degenerative changes occur throughout the vestibular apparatus; loss of hair cells, otoconia, nerve fibers and Purkinje cells (cerebellum).
- Degenerative changes also affect the visual and proprioceptive inputs.
- Degenerative changes of the CNS, such as brainstem and cerebellar atrophy and white matter changes.
- Coexiting medical conditions, such as Parkinson's disease or diabetes mellitus with peripheral neuropathy.
- Medications used for comorbid conditions may also cause dizziness.

Management Old Age Dizziness

- Identifying and managing individual contributory factors like changing antihypertensive drugs and cataract surgery, etc.
- *Physiotherapy:* Stimulate central compensation, strengthen sensory inputs and strategies to improve balance and prevent falls.
- Pharmacotherapy.

DIZZINESS IN CHILDREN

- It is less common complaint in children than adults.
- Assessment of a dizzy child is challenging because child is unable to communicate properly.
- The child's symptoms may be attributed to behavioral problems or clumsiness.
- Many of the causes of vertigo in adults can also affect children. These include BPPV, vestibular neuronitis, perilymph fistulas, traumatic labyrinthine injuries and migraine.
- Bilateral vestibulopathy can occurs secondary to ototoxicity or bacterial meningitis.
- Motion sickness, however, does not affect children below the age of two.
- The diagnosis and management of a dizzy child will frequently need the expertise of a pediatrician.

Diagnoses of vertigo from clinical presentation are given in **Table 3.1**.

DIZZINESS IN PREGNANCY

- It is often due to hyperemesis gravidarum, which occurs mainly in the first trimester.
- Auditory or vestibular complaints in pregnancy can be obstetric (antiphospholipid syndrome) or otologic (Ménière's disease, acoustic neuroma).
- If vestibular cause is suspected, then further assessment by an otologist is required.
- Administration of any drugs during this period should be done with caution due to fetal risk of teratogenicity.

POST-TRAUMATIC VERTIGO

Vertigo or dizziness following trauma can be due to a number of causes secondary to head injury or a whiplash injury to the neck.

Table 3.1 Determining the causes of vertigo from clinical presentations

Clinical features	Possible causes
• Episode of vertigo lasting for hours, fluctuating and progressive sensorineural hearing loss and tinnitus	Ménière's disease
• Episodes of vertigo lasting less than 1 minute that are brought by rapid head movement in a nonaxial plane	Benign positional vertigo
• Vertigo and hearing loss following bacterial or viral infection	Labyrinthitis
• Hearing loss and vertigo following injury to the ear or barotraumas (such as from recent air travel or diving)	Perilymph fistula
• Acute onset of vertigo that lasts days to weeks, nausea and vomiting	Vestibular neuronitis
• Vertigo accompanied by diplopia, dysarthria, dysphagia, drop attacks, paresthesia and loss of motor function	Brainstem ischemic or infarction
• Vertigo and dysdiadochokinesia	Cerebellar stroke
• Vertigo and other neurological symptoms that suggest multiple sclerosis	Multiple sclerosis
• Asymmetric sensorineural hearing loss, imbalance particularly in the dark, vertigo (rare), hypoesthesia, facial paralysis (rare)	Acoustic neuroma
• Vertigo episodes lasting for hours with no significant auditory symptoms; personal or strong family history of migraine	Migrainous vertigo

- *Benign paroxysmal positional vertigo:* It is usually by canalolithiasis of the posterior semicircular canal. It can be bilateral, with one ear more severely affected compared to the other.
- *Acute labyrinthine failure:* It occurs from transverse fracture of otic capsule which results in hearing loss and severe vertigo. Clinical features are similar to that of vestibular neuritis.

- *Perilymph fistula:* Leakage of perilymph from the round window or oval window. It usually is due to subluxation of the stapes into the inner ear.
- *Acute labyrinthine or brainstem concussion:* Features are similar to acute labyrinthine fracture except that there is no evidence of fracture clinically or radiologically and symptoms are transient.
- *Whiplash injury:* It is due to hyperextension of the neck following road traffic accident. It results in injury of the anterior spinal ligaments and deep cervical muscles, which contain proprioceptive nerve endings. In addition, the vertebral arteries can be injured resulting in vertebrobasilar ischemia.
- *Postconcussion syndrome:* A mild form of brain injury, which can present with a variety of symptoms, which include dizziness, headache, cognitive and behavioral changes. A diagnosis is made when the symptoms persists for more than 3 months after the injury or start within a week of the trauma.
- *Malingering:* It should be considered in patients with delayed, exaggerated or chronic symptoms without objective findings and when monetary gain or compensation is sought.

CHAPTER 4

Diagnosis of Vertigo from History

The reasons for good history taking are:
- To get a diagnosis.
- Taking a good history is a part of treatment.
- The patient feels you are interested for the problem solving.
- When we give reassurance, which hopefully we will be able to give at the end, patients are able to accept the reassurance and take comfort from it.
- To be a proper doctor.

Two important causes of failure to manage the vertigo patients:
1. Reluctance to take a good history.
2. Failure to think about pathology.

When you are taking a history you begin at the beginning.

THINGS ABOUT DIZZY SPELLS

- Are they spells or is it just one attack?
- Are they of sudden onset when they come?
- Are they associated with other symptoms such as nausea, vomiting, deafness or tinnitus?
- Do they stop suddenly or gradually?
- How is the patient between attacks?
- Ask the patient when was the last time, they were perfectly stable and free from dizziness.
- Try to get a clear, coherent and chronological history to get a right diagnosis.

ASSESS THE PROBLEM

- Find out the details of the inconvenience that the patient experiences from the dizziness.
- Start assessing the problem when the patient is coming into your consulting chamber.
- Did he walk in unaided or did he stagger in or did somebody help him in?
- How much problems interferes with his everyday life.

If we are reluctant to take the history, then there is failure to think about the pathology.

Investigations are no substitute for a good history.

Key Points Behind Good History Taking

- Begin at the beginning.
- Stay in control.
- Assess the extent of the problem.
- Investigations are no substitute.
- A good history is a part of the treatment.

HISTORY TELLS DIAGNOSIS

- History of vertigo, vomiting, tinnitus and deafness refers to Ménière's disease.
- History of vertigo during changing head position refers to BPPV.
- History of cough, cold, fever followed by vertigo and deafness refers to viral labyrinthitis.
- History of cough, cold, fever followed by vertigo but no deafness refers to vestibular neuronitis.

Onset of Vertigo

Ask is this the first attack or recurrent?

- If recurrent vertigo
  – Ménière's disease.

- Migraine.
- Hypoglycemia.
- If non-recurrent vertigo
  - Vestibular neuronitis.
  - Drug-induced.
  - Labyrinthitis.
- In case of chronic vertigo suspect
  - Brain tumor.
  - Hypertension.
  - Diabetes.
  - Head injury, etc.

Drug History

Drugs causing vertigo are
- Antiepileptic.
- Antirheumatic.
- Antihypertensive.
- Antidiabetic.
- Aminoglycosides.
- Barbiturates, etc.

Past history of head injury, surgery and fever must be asked.

Personal History

Personal history of
- Blood pressure (High or low).
- Diabetes.
- Alcohol.
- Tobacco.
- Otorrhea.
- Cervical spondylosis.
- Heart disease.
- Arthritis, etc.

The simplified approach to dizzy patients was first described by Drachmann in 1972. The dizziness can be described in four forms:

1. *Dizziness type-1 or true vertigo:*
   - It is a vestibular problem, either peripheral or central connections.
   - The patient describes spinning or a definite rotatory feeling, typically precipitated by fast head movement, getting up or lying down and even turning in bed.

2. *Dizziness type-2 or presyncope:*
   It is essentially cardiovascular and the patient feels faintness or darkness before his eyes, when upright or on getting up.
   Causes are:
   - Postural hypotension (Confirmed by checking BP in supine and standing position).
   - Vasovagal attacks.
   - Hyperventilation.
   - Low cardiac output states.

3. *Dizziness type-3:*
   - It is basically unsteadiness or incoordinates of gait or feeling of loss of balance.
   - It typically occurs when the patients stands up or walks and is worsened by uneven ground or turning.
   - It never occurs when sitting or lying in bed.

   Causes: Mostly neurological. These are:
   - Gait ataxia.
   - Parkinsonism and other extrapyramidal disorders.
   - Cerebellar ataxia.
   - Myelopathy (e.g. cervical spondylotic myelopathy).
   - Neuropathy.
   - In the elderly, it can be due to impairment of multiple sensory organs, including vision, vestibular and peripheral neuropathy as well as chronic cerebral ischemia.

4. *Dizziness type-4:*
    - It is predominantly psychogenic.
    - The patient may be vague or describe numbness or heaviness or light feeling in the head.
    - It is actually an abnormal sensation in head, not fitting into the earlier three types.

Traditional Symptomatic Approach

- True Vertigo-Vestibular—Ear problem.
- Presyncope-Cardiovascular—Medical/Cardiological problem.
- Disequilibrium-Neurological-Neuro problem.
- Nonspecific dizziness—Psychiatric–No problem.

Certain aggravating factors trigger the vertigo and are helpful for the diagnosis of specific type of vertigo (**Table 4.1**).

Associated Features Suggesting a Central Cause of Vertigo (Box 4.1)

Ds

- Diplopia.
- Dysarthria.
- Dysphagia.
- Dysphonia.
- Dysmetria.
- Dysesthesia.
- Drop attacks.
- Down-is-up distortions (room tilt illusions).

Table 4.1 Triggers often give important clue for diagnosis

Trigger	Possible diagnosis
When turning in bed	True vertigo, e.g. BPPV
When getting up suddenly	Postural hypotension
When walking or turning	Type-3 or balance disorder
When tired or stressed out	Type-4 or presyncope

Box 4.1 Indicators of central causes of vertigo

- Focal neurological symptoms/signs (Deadly Ds—diplopia, dysarthria, dysphagia)
- Ataxia out of proportion to vertigo
- Nystagmus-Pure vertical (upbeating or downbeating), direction changing or gaze evoked and other eye movement abnormalities, e.g. gaze palsy, skew deviation (vertical misalignment of the eyes)
- Sudden, severe or sustained head or neck pain

Table 4.2 Duration of the vertiginous event

Acute long duration (Peripheral)	Vestibular neuritis, labyrinthitis, labyrinthine ischemia, labyrinthine concussion
Acute long duration (Central)	Cerebellar infarct, cerebellar hemorrhage, brainstem infarct, multiple sclerosis
Recurrent long duration (Peripheral)	Autoimmune inner ear disease, Ménière's disease, vestibular neuritis (recurrent)
Recurrent long duration (Pentral)	Vertebrobasilar ischemia, multiple sclerosis, migraine
Recurrent brief duration (Peripheral)	BPPV, superior canal dehiscence
Recurrent brief duration (Central)	Cerebellar tumor, cerebellar atrophy, multiple sclerosis

Diagnosis from Duration of Vertigo (Table 4.2)

- *If it is less than a second:* This is typically motion sensitivity or a feeling of transient dizziness on sudden movement, often only in one direction. The cause is typically old unilateral vestibular deficit, migraine or psychogenic. The patient may feel the need to hold on for support suddenly.
- *Transient vertigo lasting a few second:* It is typically positional and the most common cause is BPPV. There are also central

Table 4.3 Characteristic of peripheral and central vertigo

Characteristics	Peripheral	Central
• Overall illness	Looks worse	Milder illness
• Vertigo	More	Less
• Ataxia	Less	More
• Tinnitus/deafness/ear pain	Often present	Usually absent
• Diplopia/dysarthria/ sensory or motor symptoms, Horner's syndrome	Not present	Usually present
• Nystagmus pattern	Unidirectional, horizontal, rotatory	Direction changing
• Nausea, vomiting	May be severe	Varies

causes of which migraine is quite common, but there are some rare causes like TIA, posterior fossa tumor and demyelination.

- *Transient vertigo lasting a few minutes:* It is uncommon, but we need to consider a vertebrobasilar transient ischemic attack (TIA) or migraine or psychogenic. Even if the patient does not have diplopia or dysartheria or other neurological symptom and has vertigo or vertigo with tinnitus or deafness lasting for a few minutes, we need to keep in mind the possibility of a TIA, and therefore the possibility of a dangerous stroke occurring later.
- *Short attacks of vertigo lasting minutes to hours:* It may occur in Ménière's disease, migraine, stroke or psychogenic.
- *Vertigo for days to weeks:* Seen in acute peripheral vestibulopathy, migraine, psychogenic.
- Continuous vertigo for weeks is usually psychogenic.

Peripheral vertigo and central vertigo are differentiated from certain clinical features and history **(Tables 4.3 and 4.4)**.

CLINICAL TIPS

The three most important things in the management of vertigo are History, History and History only must be for the management of vertigo.

Diagnosis of Vertigo from History

Table 4.4 Vertigo of peripheral and central origin from patient history

Peripheral	Central
• A definitive sensation of movement is present	• The vertigo is mild and more like unsteadiness
• Vertigo is severe and paroxysmal	• Vague, no specific onset or termination
• The attacks last from minutes to days	• The attacks of vertigo lasts for weeks
• Nystagmus and associated vestibular symptoms are common	• Often no apparent nystagmus
• *Presentation:* Severe rotating or spinning sensation usually with nausea and vomiting	• Imbalance, lightheadedness, disorientation
• Consciousness maintained	• Consciousness may be lost
• *Presence of systemic disorders:* Usually absent	• Often diabetes, hypertension, atherosclerosis present
• *Progress of disease:* Improves as peripheral lesions are self-limiting and central compensation takes place	• Patient usually goes downhill and symptoms increase
• *Associated features:* Aural symptoms such as deafness, tinnitus, nausea and vomiting are often present	• Neurological features such as diplopia, headache, motor/sensory loss present

VERTIGO DIAGNOSIS

- Vertigo → History and physical examination → Blood pressure (Lying and supine) → Orthostatic → Diagnosis of orthostatic hypotension.
- Vertigo → Irregular pulse → Diagnosis of cardiac arrthythmia.
- Vertigo → Abnormal neurological examination → Differential diagnosis of CVA, CNS drugs, multiple sclerosis.
- Vertigo → History of cervical spine trauma → Yes → Vertigo-induced by position change → Yes → *Diagnosis:* BPPV.
- Vertigo → History of recent viral illness → Yes → *Diagnosis:* Viral labyrinthitis.

> **Box 4.2** Vertigo with deafness
>
> *Differential diagnosis*
> - Ménière's disease
> - Labyrinthitis
> - Acoustic neuroma
> - Labyrinthine trauma
> - Perilymph fistula
> - Ototoxicity

> **Box 4.3** Vertigo without deafness
>
> - Vestibular neuronitis
> - Benign paroxysmal vertigo
> - Ototoxicity to the vestibule
> - Motion sickness

- Vertigo → *Drug history:* antibiotics, diuretics or chemotherapy → Yes → *Diagnosis:* Toxic labyrinthitis.
- Vertigo → History of trauma → Yes → Barotrauma/Head trauma → *Diagnosis:* Round window rupture (In case of Barotrauma); temporal bone trauma (In head trauma).
- Vertigo → History of hearing loss → *Differential diagnosis:* Ménière's disease, acoustic neuroma, toxic labyrinthitis, neurosyphilis **(Boxes 4.2 and 4.3)**.

CHAPTER 5

Clinical Tests for Vertigo

Before assessing a dizzy patient, it should be born in mind that the results of these tests may be affected by prior medication like vestibular suppressants, antidepressants or sedatives. It is prudent to ask the patient to stop taking any of these medications 24–48 hours prior to vestibular assessment.

Also, if the patient demonstrates any sign of neurological emergency such as brainstem stroke, then it is imperative that the whole test battery is bypassed to carry out a thorough radiological assessment and neurological consult for the same.

ROUTINE EXAMINATIONS FOR VERTIGO PATIENTS

- General examinations.
- Examine the ears.
- Examine the cranial nerves (III–XII).
- Look for the nystagmus.
- Do balance tests.
- Do positional test.
- Tests for cerebellum.

General Examination

- Blood pressure.
- Pulse rate.
- Temperature.
- Pallor.
- Postural hypotension.

> **CLINICAL TIPS**
>
> Blood pressure measured in supine position and again 1 min after the patient stands. A systolic blood pressure drop of 20 mm Hg, diastolic blood pressure decrease of 10 mm Hg, or pulse increase of 30 beats per minute is indicative of orthostatic hypotension.

Examination of the Pinna and External Auditory Canal

The pinna and external auditory canal should be thoroughly examined for any vesicles which may indicate Ramsay Hunt syndrome (it causes vertigo, deafness and facial palsy). The post-auricular area and space between the tragus and helix should be searched for any scar marks of surgical incision which may be suggestive of previous ear surgery.

Otoscopic Examination (Fig. 5.1)

It can help to identify any perforation in tympanic membrane or glomus tumor or otitis media. It is always important to rule out bacterial labyrinthitis and perilymph fistula during otoscopic examination.

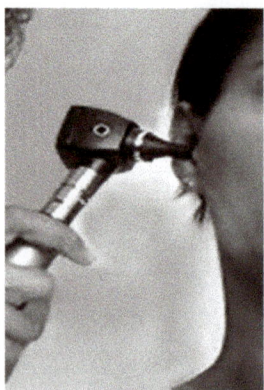

Fig. 5.1 Otoscopic examination of the ear

Tuning Fork Test

Hearing tests are must in any neuro-otological evaluation. A high-frequency hearing loss indicates a lesion in the basal turn of the cochlea, i.e. in the portion of the inner ear adjacent to the vestibular labyrinth. So, suspicion of high frequency deafness is of significant clinical relevance in balance disorder patients. Tuning fork (**Fig. 5.2**) test is used for hearing assessment at out-patient department.

Rinne's Test

- Rinne positive in normal or sensorineural hearing loss.
- Rinne negative in conductive deafness of the tested ear.
- False Rinne negative occurs in unilateral severe sensorineural deafness.

Weber's Test

- Center or equal bilaterally in normal case.
- Lateralized to one side in conductive deafness in that side and sensorineural deafness of the opposite side.

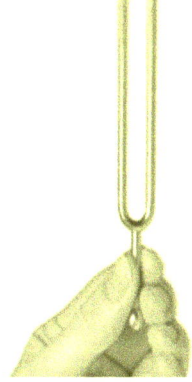

Fig. 5.2 Tuning fork

ABC Test

ABC is reduced in sensorineural deafness.

Neurological Examination

- Examination of cranial nerves at least 3rd, 4th, 5th, 6th, 7th and 9th should be done.
- Babinski's test should be done.
- Deep tendon reflexes should be checked.
- Evaluation of motor and sensory loss.
- Cerebellar function tests.

Spontaneous Nystagmus

Nystagmus is assessed by asking the patient to sit in front of the examiner. The examiner keeps moving the fingers 45 cm from the patient's eyes and moves it right, left up and down taking care not to move more than 30° from the central position to avoid gaze nystagmus.

Presence of spontaneous nystagmus indicates an organic lesion which may be peripheral (Lesion at labyrinth or 8th nerve) or central (Lesion at vestibular nuclei, brainstem or cerebellum). Peripheral vestibular nystagmus is horizontal rotatory and have both fast and slow components. Peripheral nystagmus is fatiguable but reproducible.

The following types of nystagmus may be considered to be of central nervous system origin:

- Pure vertical nystagmus.
- Direction changing/unipositional nystagmus.
- Active nystagmus without vertigo.
- *Failure of fixation:* A nystagmus generated by a central vestibular pathology often (but not always) increases in intensity when the eyes are open (i.e. optic fixation) and decreases when the eyes are closed. This is just the opposite of

Clinical Tests for Vertigo

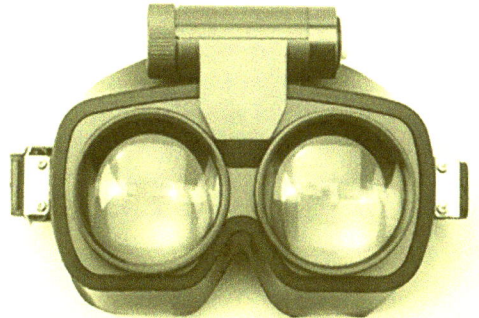

Fig. 5.3 Frenzel's glass

a peripheral vestibular lesion. Removal of optic fixation with a Frenzel's glasses (**Fig. 5.3**) may help unmask latent nystagmus.
- Dysconjugate eye movement in nystagmus, and gaze nystagmus (the patient cannot maintain conjugate eye deviation away from the midline).

Rotatory nystagmus, however is commonly associated with peripheral vestibular system disorders. Spontaneous nystagmus in peripheral vestibular disease, is an oscillating motion of both eyes that has two phases, a slow one that moves toward the side of the lesion and a quick phase that moves towards the opposite side. Therefore, this means that the slow phase indicates the side of the peripheral lesion (**Fig. 5.4**).

Central and peripheral nystagmus are differentiated by certain features are given (**Table 5.1**).

Alexander's Law

Horizontal nystagmus of peripheral origin (labyrinth or VIII nerve) obeys Alexander's law, which states the nystagmus:
- It is always in one direction irrespective of the direction of gaze.

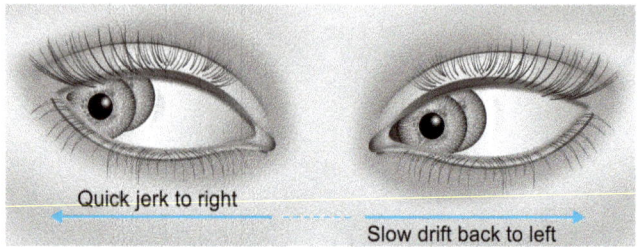

Fig. 5.4 Spontaneous nystagmus in left peripheral vestibulopathy

Table 5.1 Difference between central and peripheral nystagmus		
	Central nystagmus	*Peripheral nystagmus*
Type	Rotatory, mixed	Horizontal/vertical
Fatiguability	Not fatiguable	Fatiguable
Induction	Not possible	Possible
Latency	No latency	Present (2–20 sec)
Duration	No fixed duration	Less than 1 minute
Accompanying symptoms	CNS features	Vertigo

- Intensity of the nystagmus is greatest when looking in the direction of the fast phase.

Opsoclonus: Here the eye movements are non-rhythmic and very bizarre—the eyes moving rapidly but irregularly in all directions—horizontal, vertical, oblique or rotator. It occurs in lesions of the brainstem and cerebellum.

Ocular myoclonus: This is a pendular oscillatory movement of the eyes which occur synchronously with similar rhythmical movements of the soft palate, tongue and larynx. The cause is believed to be an advanced lesion in the dentate nucleus or its central connections with possibly a pseudohypertrophy of the inferior olivary nucleus.

Ocular bobbing: The eye shows irregular downward jerks occurring abruptly. Each downward jerk is followed by a slow return of the eyes to the mid-position. This erratic eye movement is usually binocular but may rarely be uniocular. Ocular bobbing suggests a CNS lesion.

Ocular flutter: This is a mild form of opsoclonus and consists of sudden rapid oscillatory movement of the eyes lasting for very few seconds. The patient usually complains of a sudden momentary spell of blurring of vision but it is not accompanied by a definite vertiginous sensation.

Corneal Reflex

Small cotton wool is taken and the patient is asked to look straight-forward when the examiner will touch the sclera first and then cornea. In normal condition, patient's eyes should blink on both sides on touching the cornea by cotton wool. Blinking will be absent in cerebellopontine angle pathology, e.g. acoustic neuroma. In corneal reflex, an afferent pathway (the nasociliary branch of the ophthalmic nerve, which is a branch of the trigeminal nerve), the spinal root of the trigeminal nerve which is the first synapse, the second synapse which is the nucleus of facial nerve of both sides, the efferent neural pathway (temporal branch of the facial nerve of both sides) and the effector motor organ which is the orbicularis oculi muscle of both sides (supplied by facial nerve). In this, afferent is unilateral and the efferent is bilateral pathway.

Fistula Test

It is elicited by pressing the tragus or by using siegle pneumatic speculum. Positive fistula test means that patient will complain of vertigo while performing the test and nystagmus will be directed towards opposite side.

> **CLINICAL TIPS**
>
> *Positive fistula test* implies that there is a fistula communicating middle ear and inner ear. The most common site of fistula formation is lateral semicircular canal.
>
> *False negative fistula sign:* There is fistula but the labyrinth is dead or the fistula is covered by granulation tissue or cholesteatoma mass.
>
> *False positive fistula sign:* There is no fistula but the test is positive. It is seen in early congenital syphilis where annular ligament is lax and mobile known as Hennebert's sign. It is also seen in Ménière's disease and following fenestration surgery. Tullio phenomenon is seen in labyrinthine fistula and following fenestration surgery where giddiness is produced more by loud noise rather than pressure.

Valsalva Maneuver

- Forced exhalation with closed nostril and mouth increases pressure in the middle ear through eustachian tube. It causes vertigo in some cases of perilymphatic fistulae.
- Forced exhalation with closed glottis raises intracranial pressure, which can cause dizziness in cases of superior semicircular canal dehiscence and Chiari malformations.

Standing Test

The patient will stand with eyes open, feet close together, then eyes closed and finally stand on one leg with eye closed. The patient stands for about 15–20 seconds on the left leg, followed by 15–20 seconds on the right leg. Any swaying of the body is looked for. In acute peripheral vestibular lesion, body is twisted to the side of lesion, deviation of both arms to the side of the lesion with raising of the hand on the healthy side with a tendency of falling to the side of the lesion. This typical position is called discus-thrower's position.

Walking Test

- The patient is asked to walk with feet tandem. He is also allowed to walk with the toe of the backfoot touching the heel of the frontfoot in a straight line with closed eye and eye open.
- Falling or deviation or tendency to fall is noted.
- Falling or deviating repeatedly in the same direction suggests an unilateral vestibular lesion on the side of the fall.
- A broad and wide-based gait with tendency to fall, suggests the possibility of a cerebellar pathology.
- If the patient walk backwards with feet tandem, there should be no reason to suspect any organic balance disorder.

Romberg Test

The patient will stand with feet together and arms by the side with eyes open first and then closed. If eyes open, patient can still compensate the imbalance but with eyes closed, vestibular system is at more disadvantages. In peripheral vestibular lesions, the patient sways to the side of lesion. In central vestibular lesion, patient shows instability. If patient performs this test without sway, sharpened Romberg test can be performed. In this test, patient stands with one heel in front of toes and arms folded across the chest. Inability to perform the sharpened Romberg test indicates vestibular impairment.

Unterburger's Test

The blind-folded patient is asked to extend his arms and step on the same spot alternately with each foot for 90 times in 1 min **(Fig. 5.5)**. In peripheral vestibular lesions, the patient rotates/deviates to the side of the lesion. In central vestibular lesion, the sway (i.e. the side-to-side movement while stepping) is abnormally high.

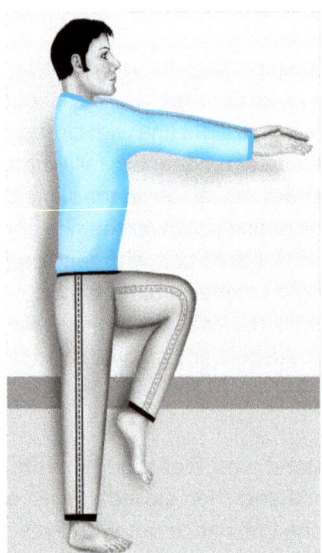

Fig. 5.5 Unterberger's test

Head Shaking Test (Fig. 5.6)

The head of the patient is grasped by the clinician and shaken rapidly and vigorously side to side for 20 times and any nystagmus is looked for. Presence of nystagmus suggests a disorder in the vestibular system, usually peripheral in nature. No nystagmus is obtained on head shaking in normal subjects. Usually, a left beating nystagmus suggests a right peripheral lesion and vice versa. Vertical nystagmus is sometimes found in lesions of the central vestibular system.

Rotation Test

The patient sits on a special chair (**Fig. 5.7**) and rotates with eyes closed 10 times in 20 seconds. The after nystagmus is measured

Clinical Tests for Vertigo

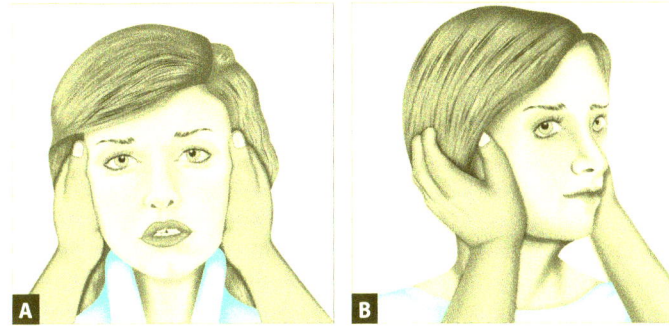

Figs 5.6A and B Head shaking test

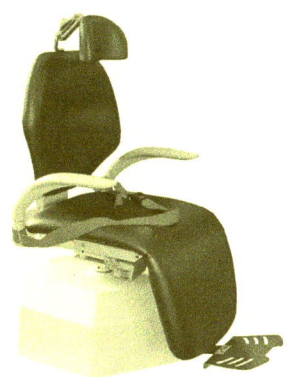

Fig. 5.7 Special chair used for rotation test

with a stopwatch, which varies from 15 to 30 seconds in a normal individual. In active labyrinth, the nystagmus will be on the opposite side of the rotation.

Positional Test (Dix-Hallpike Test)

It is done when patient complains of vertigo during change of head position.

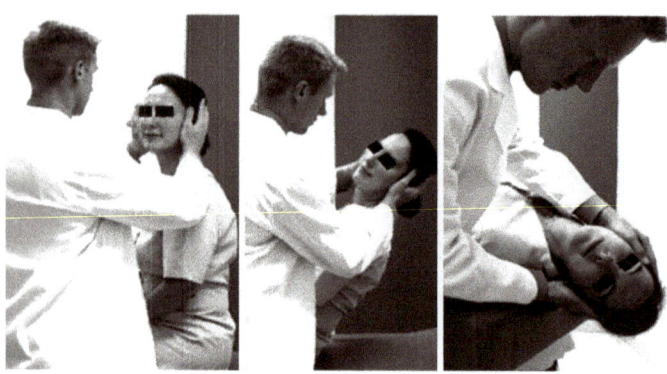

Fig. 5.8A Steps of Dix-Hallpike test

Patient sits on a couch. Examiner hold the patient's head, turn it 45° to the right and then places the patient in a supine position so that his head hangs 30° below the horizontal (**Figs 5.8A and B**). Patient's eyes are observed for nystagmus. The test is repeated with head turned to left and then again in straight head-hanging position. Four parameters of the nystagmus are observed: Latency, duration, direction and fatiguability. In BPPV, nystagmus appears after a latent period of 2–20 seconds, lasts for less than a minute and is always in one direction, i.e. towards the ear that is undermost. On repetition of the test, nystagmus may still be elicited but lasts for a shorter period. On subsequent repetitions, it disappears altogether, i.e. nystagmus is fatiguable. Patient also complains of vertigo when the head is in critical position.

In central lesions (e.g. tumors of 4th ventricle, cerebellum, temporal lobe, multiple sclerosis, vertebrobasilar insufficiency or raised intracranial tension), nystagmus is produced immediately, as soon as the head is in critical position without any latency and lasts as long as head is in that critical position. Direction of nystagmus also varies in different test positions (direction changing) and is non-fatiguable on repetition of test (**Table 5.2**).

Clinical Tests for Vertigo

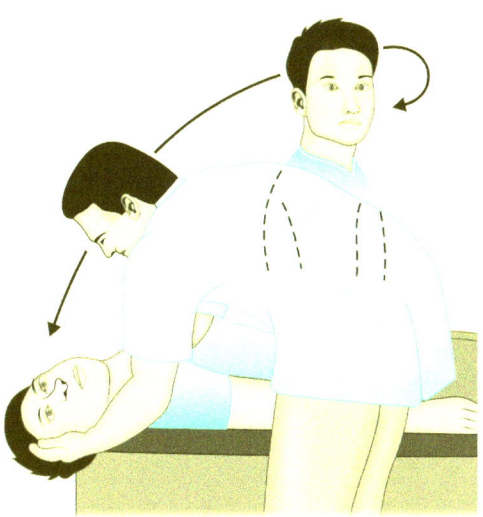

Fig. 5.8B Dix-Hallpike test

Table 5.2 Differences between peripheral and central causes of positional nystagmus

	Peripheral nystagmus	Central nystagmus
Onset	Delayed (2–20 seconds)	Immediate
Distress	Severe vertigo during nystagmus with distress	None
Fatiguability	Fatigues on repetition of the test	Does not fatigue
Duration	Less than 1 minute	More than 1 minute
Direction	Direction fixed, towards the undermost ear	Direction changing

Minimal Physical Examination in Dizzy Patients

- Check BP in supine and standing.
- Check for spontaneous nystagmus fixating a target and with fixation blocked.

> **Table 5.3** How to differentiate acute posterior fossa stroke from acute peripheral vestibulopathy?
>
> 1. *Walk the patient:* Stroke patient often cannot stand or walk unsupported
> 2. *Turns the light down:* Constricted pupil due to Horner's syndrome may appear ipsilateral to the stroke
> 3. *Check the sensation too cold on the face and extremities:* Stroke may show sensory loss for temperature on the ipsilateral face and contralateral extremities
> 4. *Test for dysdiadochokinesia:* It will affects the ipsilateral hand after a cerebellar stroke
> 5. Unilateral hearing loss can occur ipsilateral stroke and does not prove the origin of vertigo is peripheral

- Check smooth pursuit and saccadic eye movements.
- Head impulse test.
- Hallpike test.
- Check standing balance (Romberg) and check gait.
- Dynamic visual quality.

Orthostatic Hypotension

Blood pressure measured in supine position and again 1 minute after the patient stands. A systolic blood pressure drop of 20 mm Hg, diastolic blood pressure decrease of 10 mm Hg or pulse increase of 10 beats per minute is indicative of orthostatic hypotension. It is seen in cases of dehydration or autonomic dysfunction.

Clinical tips differentiating central vertigo (Posterior fossa stroke) from acute peripheral vestibulopathy are provided in **Table 5.3**.

SPECIAL VESTIBULAR TESTS

Oscillopsia Test

- This test assesses for bilateral vestibular loss as in bilateral ototoxicity.

- The patient complains of his surrounding bobbles or shakes, whenever he is in motion.
- In this test, patient is asked to read the lowest possible on a standard Snellen's chart. Then with repetitive shaking of the head in the horizontal plane, the patient is asked to read the lowest line possible for comparison. A loss of more than four lines during active head shaking is considered significant for bilateral loss.

Vestibulo-ocular Reflex Suppression

- The peripheral vestibular systems are stimulated by head movement, while the patient is asked to fix on a certain object during these movements to suppress the vestibulo-ocular reflex (VOR) thus inhibiting nystagmus. This ability to suppress the VOR is through centrally mediated smooth pursuit pathways.
- This is in essence optic fixation and implies the ability of the visual system to override labyrinthine information provided the central pathways are normal.
- Therefore, failure of VOR suppression is indicative of central pathology.

Head Impulse/Halmagyi Test

- It tests the horizontal semicircular canal.
- In this test, quick or rapid movement of head in the horizontal plane with gaze fixed in midpoint (examiners nose). A peripheral disorder will result in a corrective saccade. A right sided lesion will result in corrective saccades to the left, when the head is turned to the right.
- A normal test helps to differentiate vestibular neuritis from pseudoneuritis (stroke).

OCULOMOTOR TESTS

These tests usually assess the oculomotor nerves and their central pathologies. Abnormalities in these tests indicate a central pathology or pathology of the oculomotor nerves (III, IV and VI).

Fixation (Table 5.4)

The patient is asked to fixate on an object held straight ahead.

Smooth Pursuit (Table 5.5)

Patient is asked to follow moving target horizontally and vertically.

Saccade (Table 5.6)

Patient is asked to fix on target 20 to 30° from midpoint and quickly change between right and left or up and down. Both horizontal and vertical saccades are tested.

Table 5.4 Testing the fixation

Findings	Interpretation
Able to fixate	Normal
Pendular nystagmus	Central cause
Jerk nystagmus	Central/peripheral vestibular disorder

Table 5.5 Testing the smooth pursuit

Findings	Interpretation
Impaired asymmetrical	Central pathology
Impaired symmetrical (slow or reduced)	Central pathology/drugs/old age/fatigue

Table 5.6 Saccades findings

Findings	Interpretation
Overhooting (hypermetric)	
Undershooting (hypometric)	
Prolonged latency	
Slow latency	Central disorders
Inaccuracy	
Inability to generate	

Convergence

Patient is asked to fixate at an object in front of him the object is slowly brought to the tip of his nose. Abnormality indicative of a central pathology.

CEREBELLAR TESTS

Past-pointing

- The patient is asked to touch the examiner's finger with his index finger at different positions.
- Intention tremor and past-pointing are indicative of a cerebellar lesion on the affected side.

Rapid Alternating Movement

- Pat the palm of one hand with the palm and dorsum of the other hand alternately.
- There will be slowness of the limb on the affected side to perform the movement (Dysdiadochokinesia).

TESTS FOR UTRICULAR/OTOLITHIC DYSFUNCTION

Eye Cover Test (For Skew Deviation)

- With the patient gazing forward one eye is covered followed by the other.

- Vertical deviation of the uncovered eye with the other eye covered usually indicates a central pathology.

Ocular Tilt Reaction

- The ocular tilt reaction consists of a triad of skew deviation, ocular torsion and head tilt.
- The causes are Ménière's disease, vestibular neuritis, acoustic neuromas and strokes.
- In one side labyrinthine hypofunction, it consists of head tilt towards the lesioned labyrinth, skew deviation with the lower eye on the side of the lesion and ocular counter roll (torsional deviation of the superior poles of the eyes toward the side of the lesion).
- In normal patients, ocular torsion of the upper poles of the eyes rotates toward the higher ear.

Subjective Visual Vertical

- Injury to the otoliths or to the nerve that transmits impulses from the otoliths and other parts of the ear to the brain, judgment of vertical may be altered.
- Patients with peripheral vestibular and brainstem lesions, there is deviation of the subjective vertical.
- However, in cerebellar lesions, there is good accuracy of the subjective vertical.

Chapter 6

Investigations for Vertigo

HEMATOLOGICAL TESTS

- Full blood count.
- A raised erythrocyte sedimentation rate (ESR) may raise the suspicion of an infecting or autoimmune pathology.
- Fasting blood sugar.
- Lipid profile.
- Blood urea and serum electrolytes.
- Cardiac enzymes.
- Thyroid function test.
- Fluorescent treponemal antibody-absorption (FTA-ABS) or venereal disease research laboratory (VDRL) should be done for detecting a syphilitic infection.
- Test for rheumatoid factor, urine analysis, antinuclear antibody checks for a possible autoimmune pathology.

AUDIOLOGICAL TEST

Pure tone audiometry (PTA).

RADIOLOGICAL TESTS

- CT scan.
- MRI.
- Functional MRI (f-MRI).
- Positron emission tomography (PET).
- Single photon emission computerized tomography (SPECT).

High Resolution CT Scan and MRI Scan Help to Rule Out Retrocochlear Pathology

- A unilateral or asymmetrical sensorineural hearing loss is an indication for imaging to exclude a tumor of the VII cranial nerve. Gadolinium MRI is the imaging of choice.
- Consider MRI for suspecting cerebrovascular disease.
- MRI or conventional angiography of the posterior fossa vasculature may be useful in diagnosing vasculature causes of vertigo such as vertebrobasilar insufficiency, thrombosis of the labyrinthine artery, anterior or posterior inferior cerebellar artery insufficiency and subclavial steal syndrome.
- CT scans can be used, if MRI is contraindicated or in suspected cases of cholesteatoma.

The structural imaging like CT scans or MRIs show abnormalities, only when there is any structural defect of any of constituents of the balance system, viz any tumor or bleeding/infarction of the tissues, etc. But the balance problems are rarely caused by such structural changes, they are usually a result of subtle functional disorders, and hence it is functional imaging such as f-MRI, PET and SPECT that are more relevant and more informative in disorders of the balance system. A normal CT scan/MRI does not rule out a balance disorder.

GLYCEROL TEST

- It is an useful test for Ménière's disease.
- Glycerol is a dehydrating agent. When it is given orally, it reduces endolymphatic pressure and thus causes an improvement of hearing.
- Glycerol (1.5 mL/kg) is given to patient with an equal amount of water and a little flavoring agent or lemon juice.
- Audiogram and speech discrimination scores are recorded before and 1–2 hours after ingestion of glycerol.

- An improvement of 10 decibel in two or more adjacent octaves or gain of 10% in discrimination score makes the test positive. There is also improvement in tinnitus and in the sense of fullness in the ear.
- This test has a diagnostic and prognostic value. Presently, this test is combined with electrocochleography.

SPECIAL VESTIBULAR INVESTIGATIONS

Assessment of Vestibulo-ocular Reflex

- Electronystagmography (ENG).
- Videonystagmography (VNG).

Assessment of Vestibulospinal Reflex

- Craniocorpography (CCG).
- Computerized dynamic posturography (CDP).

Electronystagmography (ENG)

- It is the most popular vestibular function test.
- It is a test for assessing the integrity of the vestibule-ocular and allied reflex systems like the smooth pursuit system, the optokinetic system and saccadic systems.
- ENG is expressed in butterfly chart (**Fig. 6.1**).
  Normal = 0, Hypoactivity = 1 and Hyperactivity = 2.

Videonystagmography (VNG)

- It is a computerized process of the electronically scanning the eye movements through small high resolution charged coupled device (CCD) sensor cameras and then processing the video images digitally to record and document the eye movement and compute them for analyzing the different parameters like speed of slow phase, culmination frequency, etc.

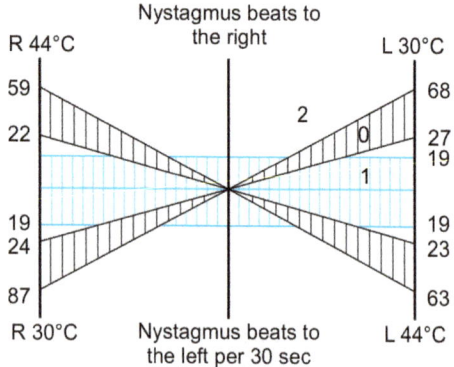

Fig. 6.1 Claussen butterfly chart

- One of the major advantages of VNG over ENG is that VNG can record rotatory eye movement (in BPPV) that is not possible by ENG.

Craniocorpography

- It tests the vestibule-spinal system.
- It consists of photographically recording the patient's head and body movements as he or she performs the Unterburger's stepping test and the Romberg's test.

Computerized Dynamic Posturography (CDP)

- It is a series of vestibule-spinal tests for quantitatively assessing balance function in different set-ups which simulate conditions encountered in our day-to-day life.
- The tests of CDP help us in identifying the system at fault and in analyzing the integrity of the CNS for the proper maintenance of balance.

Investigations for Vertigo

Vestibular Evoked Myogenic Potentials (VEMP)

- Saccule is the source of VEMP.
- If saccule is damaged, then VEMP is absent.
- This investigation evaluates the inferior vestibular nerve which innervates the saccule and posterior semicircular canal.
- The saccule is sensitive to sound stimulation results in a reflex mechanism which relaxes the sternocleidomastoid muscle.
- In this test, clicks or tonal stimuli (sound) is introduced into one ear and sternocleidomastoid electromyography is recorded with electrodes.
- It is useful in the diagnosis of superior semicircular canal dehiscence, vestibular neuritis (when there is inferior vestibular nerve involvement), bilateral vestibular loss and monitoring intratympanic gentamycin therapy for Ménière's disease.

Caloric Test

If water at 30°C and 44°C (i.e. 7°C below and above normal body temperature) is run into the ear canal (**Fig. 6.2**), nystagmus is produced in the normal persons with a healthy labyrinth. The nystagmus lasts for about 2 minutes from beginning of stimulation. If the time of nystagmus lasts for less than average, it is called as canal paresis. Directional preponderance of nystagmus either to right or to left is also a finding. Both canal paresis and directional preponderance may occur either singly or in combination. Canal paresis will be present in majority of patients with Ménière's disease, vestibular neuronitis and acoustic neuroma. In the lesion of posterior part of the temporal lobe, directional preponderance will be seen towards the side of the lesion.

Optokinetic Test

Patient is asked to follow a series of vertical stripes on a drum moving first from right to left and then from left to right.

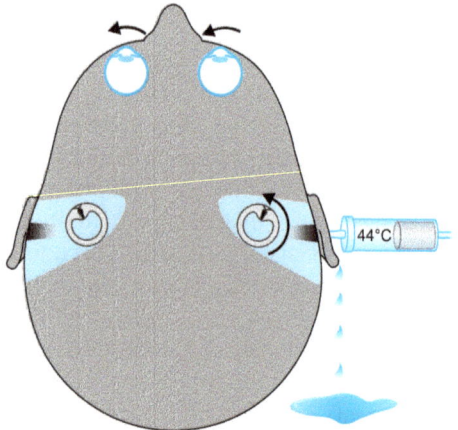

Fig. 6.2 Caloric test

Normally, it produces nystagmus with slow component in the direction of moving stripes and fast component in the opposite direction. Optokinetic abnormalities are seen in brainstem and cerebellar hemisphere lesions. Thus, this test is useful to diagnose a central lesion.

Electrocochleography

- Electrocochleography (ECochG) is a variant of brainstem audio-evoked response (ABR) where sound stimulation is provided but the recording electrode is placed as close to the cochlea, near the tympanic membrane or transtympanic.
- Action potential (AP) is the compound action potential of the auditory nerve.
- Summating potential (SP) is the response of the cochlea to sound stimulation.
- It is used for diagnosis of Ménière's disease where SP/AP ratio is more than 0.5.

Rotatory Chair

- This assesses both horizontal semicircular canals bilaterally and it is considered the gold standard for bilateral peripheral vestibular loss.
- It is somewhat similar to the caloric test which assesses the function of the horizontal semicircular canal.
- The rotational chair testing has a sensitivity of 71% for diagnosis peripheral vestibulopathies, as opposed to only 31% sensitivity for caloric testing/ENG.
- Used for the diagnosis of peripheral vestibular disorders, bilateral vestibular loss, monitoring patients undergoing pharmacologic vestibular ablation for Ménière's disease/syndrome and for medicolegal purposes.

CONDITIONS REQUIRING URGENT NEUROIMAGING (CT/MRI)

- Sudden onset of vertigo (seconds) that persists and not provoked by position.
- Association with deafness but no typical Ménière's history.
- Association with new onset (occipital) headache.
- Acute vertigo with normal head impulse test.
- Associated with central neurological signs such as severe gait and truncal ataxia.

CHAPTER 7

Treatment of Vertigo

OBJECTIVE OF TREATMENT

- Correct the cause (Not merely suppress the symptom).
- Promote vestibular compensation.
- Drugs that depress the CNS jeopardize the central compensatory mechanism and inhibit vestibular compensation.
- Peripheral vestibular disorders are usually self-limiting.
- Vertigo/imbalance and psychogenic disorders are comorbid conditions; the psychogenic part needs effective management.
- Cognitive disorders are very common in balance disorder patients; correction of the concomitant cognitive deficit yields better treatment outcomes.
- Neurotropic agents/antioxidants/cognition-enhancing drugs have a positive role in the management of balance disorders.

PRINCIPLES OF MANAGEMENT OF VERTIGO

- Treat the cause.
- Suppress the vestibular system.
- Suppress the emotional reaction.
- Encourage the compensation.
- Surgery.
- Accept the problem.

Treat the Cause
- Perform Epley maneuver in case of benign paroxysmal positional vertigo (BPPV).
- Some give steroids in acute vertigo.
- In Ménière's disease, treat the cause. But the sad thing is that the cause of Ménière's disease is not known.

Suppress the Vestibular System
This is done by giving vestibular sedatives.

Suppress the Emotional Reaction
- Many patients feel miserable.
- Many patients feel it is the end of the world.
- Even some think there may be the brain tumor.
- Some think there may occur stroke.
- So we should reassure these patients that they are not having a stroke, that it will settle down, that it is not going to go on forever and that they are not going to die.

Encourage Compensation
- We need to encourage compensation.
- If we do nothing in a young person following a destructive lesion, they will get better.
- If patient is older, they need active support and instruction in vestibular rehabilitation.

Three Simple Exercises for Compensation
1. The first, move the head from side-to-side and up-and-down. We should explain the patient that initially these exercises will make them feel worse for few days.
2. The second exercise is to get the patient to put his arms out in front, to fix his eyes on his thumb nails and just move the head

from side to side, keeping the eyes fixed on to his thumb nails. And then do the same, up and down.
3. The third exercise is rather similar. With outstretched arms, look at the thumb nails and just swing around from side to side.

Generally, we advise these exercises for just 5 minutes, 4 times a day. Initially, this makes them dizzy, but if they keep doing them, the exercises stop making them feeling dizzy. And when that has happened, the central compensation has occurred.

The Cowthorne-Cooksey exercises are also excellent.

Surgery

This is indicated very rarely in vertigo.

Disturbances in Labyrinth

Stimulation:
- Benign positional vertigo rarely requires surgery.
- Labyrinthine fistula, usually due to cholesteatoma requires surgery.
- Dehiscent superior semicircular canal, most of these patients once they have this situation explained to them, feel much better about it and usually do not require surgery.

Incomplete Destruction

Causes
- Trauma.
- Inflammatory diseases.
- Vascular diseases.

Since, we have got a better understanding of vestibular rehabilitation, surgery is almost never required in incomplete destruction of labyrinth.

Irritation of labyrinth

Causes
- Chronic suppurative otitis media (CSOM).
- Perilymph fistula.

Intermittent Failure of Labyrinth

Causes
- Delayed hydrops.
- Ménière's disease.

Surgery is only very rarely indicated in intermittent failure of the labyrinth in delayed hydrops and Ménière's disease.

Accepting the Problem

The 6th principle of management is accepting the problem. For example, if we got somebody particularly an elderly person with vestibular inadequacy, there is no point in keeping on doing investigations and keeping on trying other drugs. Sometimes, drugs will make them worse. Here, we should reassure them that there is no serious underlying problem, give them advice on living with their problem, with their unsteadiness, encourage them to use a walking stick and discharge them. Do not keep bringing them back.

About 90% of the vertigo patients will get good result by above six principles.

We will discuss treatment of different causes of vertigo step by step.

We already classified the vertigo
- Sensation of rotation
    1. Episodic (seconds/hours).
    2. Prolonged (weeks).

- Sensation of unsteadiness
    1. Episodic (seconds/hours to days).
    2. Prolonged (weeks to months/forever).

ROTATORY VERTIGO

Short-lived Spinning

- The underlying pathology for the episodic spinning dizziness, which lasts for seconds is largely labyrinthine stimulation.
- Occasionally, it is depression but usually stimulation.

Causes of Short-lived Spinning/Episodic Rotatory Vertigo (seconds)

- Benign positional vertigo.
- Labyrinthine fistula.
- Caloric effect.
- Alternobaric vertigo.
- Vertebrobasilar insufficiency.
- Dehiscent superior semicircular canal.

Benign positional vertigo:
- Most common example of short-lived spinning.
- Treatment is the Epley maneuver.
- Drugs have no part to play in benign positional vertigo.
- Explain to them that every time they experience dizziness they are one step nearer to the end of dizziness.

Labyrinthine fistula:
- If we exert the pressure in the external auditory canal or middle ear, this conveys pressure through the vestibular system and this moves to the ampullary cupula. Patient experiences short-lived but very severe spinning dizziness.
- The most common cause is the cholesteatoma.
- The treatment is surgery.

Caloric effect:
- Caloric stimulation gives short-lived spinning dizziness.
- The dizziness wears off once the caloric effect is worn-off.

Alternobaric vertigo:
- It is a rare condition.
- It occurs in the jet fighter pilot or in the diver.
- There is sudden pressure change within the middle ear, which will be transmitted into the inner ear and cause sudden short-spinning dizziness which lasts only seconds.

Vertebrobasilar insufficiency:
- Do not diagnose vertebrobasilar insufficiency on the evidence of vertigo alone.
- You need some other symptoms for diagnosis such as double vision, blurring of vision, dysarthria and numbness.

Dehiscent superior semicircular canal:
- Tullio phenomenon is present.
- There is siphoning-off of the sound energy which should be going into the cochlea.
- Very rarely does this require surgery but sometimes it does.

EPISODIC FOR HOURS

Ménière's Disease

- The most common example is Ménière's disease. The hearing loss and tinnitus should be fluctuating in association with the vertigo which should be rotatory, episodic, usually incapacitating. It is usually associated with nausea and sometimes vomiting, of sudden onset and relatively sudden cessation with, at least in the early stages, the patient perfectly well between attacks.
- If there is no hearing loss, tinnitus and nausea or vomiting, only dizziness for more than 24 hours, do not diagnose Ménière's disease.

- We cannot influence the course of Ménière's disease. We can treat the acute attack by labyrinthine sedatives. We cannot influence the next attack though we can reassure the patient that it is nothing serious.
- Surgery for Ménière's disease is very rarely indicated.
- Endolymphatic sac surgery has not much helpful in disease process.
- Gentamycin injection is a treatment.
- Labyrinthectomy can be done, but it destroys all the inner ear.
- Vestibular nerve section is an useful procedure.

Syphilitic Labyrinthitis

- Routine test is fluorescent treponemal antibody (FTA).
- The big difference between syphilitic labyrinthitis and Ménière's disease is that the disease course tends to be more rapidly progressive, and secondly that the other ear tends to be involved much earlier than one would expect in Ménière's disease.

PROLONGED ROTATORY

- The dizziness lasts for weeks and rotatory vertigo never lasts for longer than three weeks.
- This is due to some destruction of the labyrinth or the vestibular nerve.
- They have incapacitating vertigo with vomiting.
- Spinning dizziness gradually improves but is followed by unsteadiness which will improve.
- The best way to make them normal is rehabilitation exercises.
- Vestibular neuronitis is the most obvious and most common example.
- Trauma during ear surgery or labyrinthectomy or vestibular nerve section can also produce prolonged rotatory vertigo.
- Vascular lesions will also cause prolonged rotatory vertigo.

- Metastatic deposits in the cerebellum pontine angle can also cause for prolonged vertigo. This is secondary from a breast cancer. These type patients are terminally ill and very often die undiagnosed.

UNSTEADINESS

Short-lived
- The unsteadiness is usually a problem somewhere within the system and so exclusively in the ear.
- This is due to a physiological overload of the central processing.
- It can occur when there is abnormal input which may be visual and this includes looking down from a height where the input is abnormal and the central processor has difficulty dealing with it, causing a feeling of unsteadiness. Abnormal inputs can also from the cervical spine doing the same thing.

Unsteadiness for Hours
- The most common cause is the self-inflicted drug alcohol. But it can also occur from other drugs.
- Motion sickness is an another cause.
- Perilymph fistula is also a cause.
- Active chronic otitis media is also a cause unsteadiness which will settle down, if we treat the otitis media.
- Hyperventilation is another cause of this unsteadiness which lasts for a variable period of time.
- Psychogenic cause may be due to nervous tension or may be due to malingering.

Prolonged Unsteadiness
- Unsteadiness lasts for weeks to months.
- This is due to vestibular inadequacy.

- The most common cause is aging.
- The prolonged unsteadiness can again occur from drugs, the metabolic effect for example of anticonvulsants and when we stop the drug they get back to normal.
- The ototoxic drug is also a cause where the damage is permanent. They have lost their vestibular function and patient will improve by labyrinthine exercises. Labyrinthine sedative drugs will often make them worse. Labyrinthine exercises will help them but remain always with a certain degree of unsteadiness.
- Central nervous system lesions can also cause unsteadiness.
- *Floating patients:* These are patients who frequently describe the floating sensation and they can go on for years. They never have to cancel any social event, they can always do what they plan to do but they just feel that they are floating. All tests are normal. The treatment is to reassure them and there are many instances when they will eventually settle down.
- In case of infected mastoid cavity, patient go on for a long period of time feeling unsteady. They settle down with the cavity infection and then feel better.

Treatment of Peripheral Vertigo

- Pharmacotherapy.
- Adoptive exercise.
- Surgery.

Pharmacotherapy

Drug therapy for vertigo is used for symptomatic treatment and to treat the underlying disorder.

The common specific peripheral vestibular disorders amenable to pharmacotherapy are:
- Ménière's disease.
- Vestibular neuritis.

- Autoimmune inner disorder.
- Infective labyrinthitis.

The common specific central vestibular disorders amenable to pharmacotherapy are:
- Migraine-related vertigo.
- Epileptic vertigo.
- Multiple sclerosis.
- Vertebrobasilar insufficiency.

The causative factors for the balance disorder in the non-specific central/peripheral vestibular disorder patients are usually one or more of the followings:
- Hypoxia in the brain and/or inner ear.
- Metaboilc disorders.
- Degenerative changes in the sensory epithelium of the inner ear and in the neuronal tissues of the brain.
- Neurotransmitter dysfunction (hyperactivity/hypoactivity of neurotransmitter).
- Psychophysiologic disorders.

CLINICAL TIPS

The aim of drug therapy in nonspecific balance disorders should be directed to correct the possible etiologies and care being taken to ensure that the patient gets symptomatic relief from the vertigo/vomiting and lastly the vestibular compensatory mechanism is not inhibited in any way.

An ideal anti-vertigo drug should
- Control vertigo/instability and nausea/vomiting.
- Enhance cerebral and inner-ear blood flow.
- Free from side effects such as drowsiness, central nervous system (CNS) depression, extrapyramidal symptoms.
- Not depress vestibular compensatory mechanism.

Treatment of Acute Vertigo Attack (Table 7.1)

- Patients with acute severe vertigo appear ill due to the vertigo and accompanying nausea and vomiting. It is considered as an

Table 7.1 Drugs for acute attack/symptomatic treatment

Vestibular sedatives	Benzodiazepines	Diazepam, Lorazepam
	Antihistamines, anticholinergics	Meclizine, dimenhydrinate, scopalamine
Antiemetics	Metoclopramide, phenothiazines	Prochlorperazine (stemetil)

emergency and medical care is urgently required. If the vertigo does not subside rapidly, it may results in hospitalization of the patient.
- An acute and severe episode of vertigo, regardless of the underlying cause, will usually settle by itself within 24–48 hours due to the effect of brainstem compensation.
- During the acute phase, supportive measures, bed rest, vestibular suppressants **(Box 7.1)** and antiemetics **(Box 7.2)** should be used to provide symptomatic relief.
- Genenrally, a combination of vestibular suppressants and an antiemetic is used. The major classes of vestibular suppressants include antihistamines, benzodiazepines and anticholinergics.
- There is evidence to show that use of vestibular suppressants can delay the compensatory mechanism of brainstem and prolong the symptoms of vertigo. In addition, these medications carry risks of side effects. Therefore, prolonged use of symptomatic medications for acute vertigo is best avoided, especially if a specific treatable cause is identified.
- When acute attack subsided, then specific treatment is done for specific diagnosis **(Table 7.2)**.
- Adjunctive treatment are also useful for controlling associated symptoms **(Table 7.3)**.

Commonly used drugs in vertigo
- Cinnarizine (Calcium-channel blocker).
- Beta-histine (Vasodilator).

Box 7.1 Drugs for controlling vertigo

- Prochlorperazine
- Dimenhydrinate
- Meclizine
- Cinnarizine
- Beta-histine

Box 7.2 Drugs for controlling nausea/vomiting

- Domperidone
- Trifluopromazine
- Metoclopramide
- Promethazine
- Ondansetron

Table 7.2 Disease specific drugs

Vestibular neuritis	Steroids	Prednisolone
Ménière's disease	Diuretics, beta-histine, calcium channel blocker	Hydrochlorothiazide Flunarizine, cinnarezine
Chronic vestibulopathy in elderly	Piracetam	

Table 7.3 Adjunctive treatment

Psychiatric	SSRI (Selective serotonin reuptake inhibitor) Tricyclic antidepressants	Fluoxetine Amitryptilline
Complementary	Ginkobiloba	

- Prochlorperazine for acute vertigo (It might precipitate extrapyramidal symptoms).

Most of the vertigo patients always remain tense and anxious. Hence, drugs like diazepam or alprazolam are preferred as adjuvant therapy.

When diagnosis is viral or bacterial labyrinthitis antiviral and broad-spectrum antibiotics must be administered.

Anticoagulants are given when it is suspected to be of thrombotic nature.

Intratympanic injection of gentamycin is preferred for advance Ménière's disease when hearing is lost but vertigo persisting.

Circulatory Mechanism of Vertigo

Increased circulatory resistance and increased blood viscosity leads to reduced microcirculation and reduced blood supply of brain and labyrinth leading to vestibular function and vertigo. Increased circulatory resistance takes place as red blood cells (RBCs) loss their flexibility due to entry of calcium ion into them. Dimension of blood vessels through which RBCs run is 3 micron while the size of RBC is 8 micron. Bigger size RBCs can run freely through small size blood vessels because they are highly flexible. If calcium ion entry into RBC, it makes them rigid. Drugs like cinnarizine (calcium-channel blocker) and beta-histine (vasodilator) are mostly useful for peripheral vertigo control as they both increase the labyrinthine circulation effectively.

Another possible cause of peripheral vertigo is abnormal firing of vestibular nuclei. Beta-histine regulates this firing activity by blocking the H3 receptors.

Contraindications of Beta-histine

- Bronchial asthma.
- Peptic ulcer.
- Pheochromocytoma.
- Concurrent use of antihistamines.

Side effect: Cinnarizine is mildly sedating drug and not liked by many ambulatory patients.

Dosage:
- Cinnarizine—25 mg tid or 75 mg OD.
- Beta-histine—8 mg tid for mild vertigo. 16 mg tid or 24 mg BD for moderate-to-severe vertigo.

MEDICATIONS IN CENTRAL VERTIGO

- Migraine-related vertigo/migraine associated vertigo
  - Migraine associated vertigo is the second most common cause of vertigo and affects almost 1% of the entire population.
  - Along with vertigo, patient presents with episodic throbbing headaches, usually unilateral accompanied by other symptoms (nausea, vomiting, photophobia or phonophobia and may be preceded by aura).
  - The duration of vertigo is usually minutes to hours, and vertigo often occurs independently of headaches.

  Treatment
  - Migraine prophylaxis, migraine-abortive medications and vestibular exercises for vertiginous migraines.
  - Prophylaxis for migraine mainly include beta-blockers, calcium channel-blockers (CCB) and tricyclic antidepressants (TCA).
  - Beta-blockers act as first line therapy in the management of migraine. They might act by decreasing prostaglandin production.
  - CCBs such as flunarizine may reduce migraine prodromes, the frequency of migraine attacks and also decrease the severity and possibility the duration of these attacks.
  - TCAs such as nortriptyline prevent migraine headaches by altering the neurotransmitters, norepinephrine and serotonin that the nerves of the brain use to communicate with one another.
  - *Migraine diet:* Avoid excessive caffeine (>2 cups of coffee/day), monosodium glutamate, chocolate, red wine and aged cheese.
- Acute vertigo caused by a cerebellar or brainstem stroke is treated with vestibular suppressants medication and minimal head movement for first few days. As soon as tolerated,

medication should be tapered and vestibular rehabilitation exercises should be initiated.
- Consider thrombolytic therapy for acute ischemic stroke only after thorough evaluation and consultation with neurologists.
- Lethargic patients or those with altered level of consciousness require vigilance and close supervision, including direct visual, ECG and pulse oximetry monitoring.
- Consider emergent interventions to minimize edema and brainstem compression in patients with altered consciousness and a deteriorating course in the emergency department. Hemorrhage or edema of posterior fossa can lead to rapid compression and compromise of vital medullary functions, obstructive hydrocephalus or herniations of the medullary tonsils.
- Do not administer anticoagulant medicine including aspirin until intracranial hemorrhage has been ruled out by imaging.
- Invasive actions may include endotracheal intubation to protect the airway, control breathing and allow therapeutic hyperventilation.
- Consider elevating the head of the bed, performing diuresis with mannitol or furosemide and administering dexamethasone.

PARTICLE REPOSITIONING AND EXERCISES FOR BPPV

Epley Maneuver (Fig. 7.1)

Patient with right posterior canal BPPV.

Step 1: Make the patient sit on the examination table with eyes open and head turned 45° to the right. Support the patient's head as the patient lies back quickly from a sitting to supine position, ending with the head hanging 20° off the end of the examination table.

Treatment of Vertigo

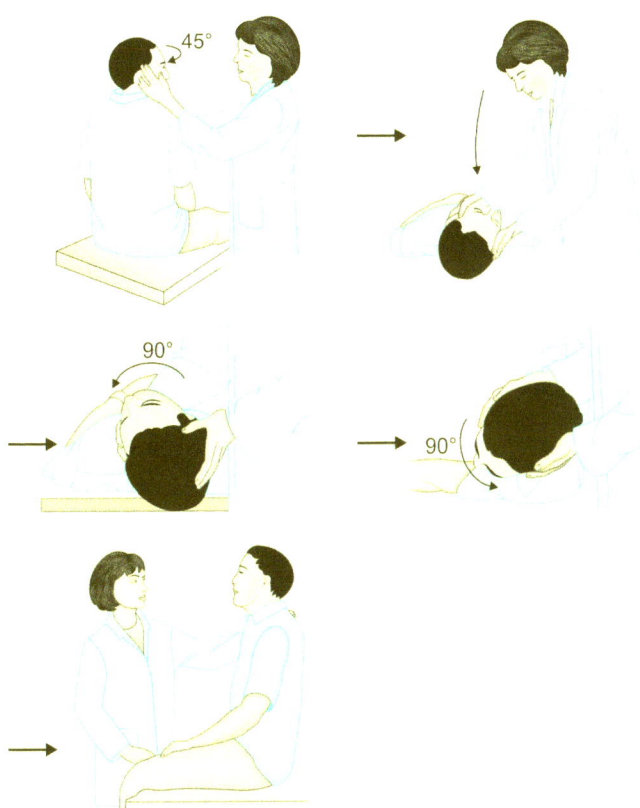

Fig. 7.1 Steps in Epley maneuver

Step 2: Turn the patient's head 90° to the left side and let the patient remains in this position for 30 sec. Turn the patient's head an additional 90° to the left while the patient rotates his or her body 90° in the same direction. Let the patient remains in this position for 30 sec.

Step 3: The patient is then made to sit up slowly with the neck flexed.

The procedure may be repeated on either side until the patient experiences relief of symptoms.

Brandt-Daroff Exercise (Fig. 7.2)

Patient with right posterior canal BPPV

Step 1: Sit upright on the side of the bed and turns the head 45° towards the healthy side.

Step 2: Patient tilts the body on the side of the affected side (right), so that the head touches the bed but the nose is pointed 45° towards the roof. Patient stays in this position for 30 sec.

Step 3: Patient sits up head straight and maintains that position for 30 sec.

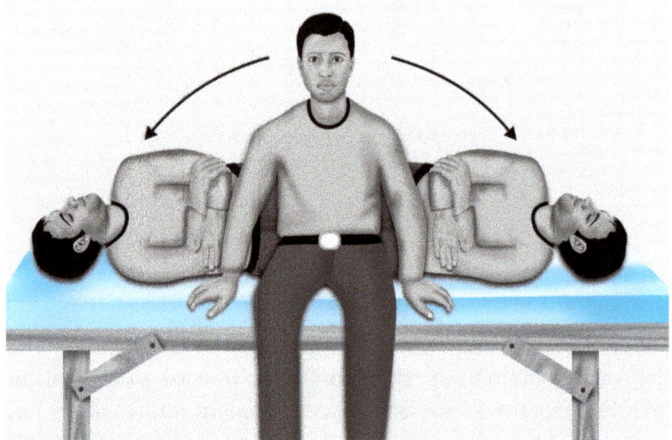

Fig. 7.2 Brandt-Daroff exercise

Step 4: The patient then lies down on the other side with the head touching the bed and nose turned 45° towards the roof.

Semont (Liberatory) Maneuver

Patient with left posterior canal BPPV.

Step 1: Patient sits at the side of the examination table and the head is turned 45° towards the healthy side (right side).

Step 2: The patient is then made to lie down very rapidly towards the side of the diseased ear such that the head hangs about 15° below the horizontal, i.e. the head is moved by 105° from the sitting position. The patient's head is kept in this position for 30 sec.

Step 3: The patient is swung by 195° to the other side, i.e. towards the side of unaffected ear and placed in such a way that the nose points downwards. The head is maintained in this position for 30 sec.

Vestibular Rehabilitation Therapy (VRT)

The head/body/eye movement exercises induce compensation by 3 mechanism, viz. adaptation, habituation and compensation. So, the exercises can be broadly divided into three groups viz. The Adaptation exercises, the Habituation exercises and the Compensation exercises according to their mechanism of action.
1. Adaptation is achieved by some exercises in the schedule of the Cawthrone-Cooksey exercises, e.g. gaze stabilization exercise. It helps the patient with peripheral vestibular disorder to adapt to the changed vestibular scenario by retaining the vestibulo-ocular reflex to stabilize images of moving objects in the fovea. In the gaze stabilization exercise, the patient is asked to follow with the eyes (without moving the head), the movement of a small rubber ball that the patient throws from one hand to the other repeatedly over the head.

Other gaze stabilization exercises are for example throwing a ball to the wall repeatedly and catching it and at the same time, following the movement of the ball with the eyes. The gaze stabilization exercises retain the extraocular muscles and re-caliberates the vestibulo-ocular reflex such that in spite of a vestibular malfunction, images of moving objects can be kept fixed in the fovea by an accurate and coordinated movement of the eyes.

2. Habituation exercises help patients of peripheral vestibular disorder by conditioning the brain through repeatedly exposure of the balance system to erroneous or mismatched sensory input. These mismatched sensory inputs induce small tolerable spells of vertigo to which the brain gets used to, so that minor vertiginous sensations are not bothersome to the patient.

   Repeatedly moving the head in the Y-axis, i.e. in the pitch plane or in the X-axis, i.e. the yaw plane stimulates the semicircular canals which inform the CNS that the subject is moving. The patient does this exercise sitting securely on the stool. So the proprioceptors inform the brain that there is no movement. When these conflicting informations (sensory mismatch/conflict) reach the CNS, the CNS is confused and it cannot reflexly generate the requisite motor output resulting in vertigo. These minor spells of vertigo, induced by erroneous or mismatched sensory input, help in habituating the balance disorder patient by conditioning the brain.

3. The compensation or substitution exercises help the patient to enhance the visual and proprioceptive inputs so that the deficit of vestibular input is counter-balanced. If one of the input systems is deficient or abnormal, the balance system can be trained to rely more on the other input system, e.g. the visual and proprioceptive systems to maintain balance. The visual and proprioceptive systems substitute for the deficient vestibular input.

Walking up and down a flight of stairs and some of the eye movement exercises are meant to sensitize the proprioceptive and visual input systems and retain the balance system to rely more on proprioceptive and visual inputs rather than on the defective vestibular input. The back movement and neck movement exercises are believed to increase spinal input to the balance system. The spinal afferent input to the vestibular nucleus is believed to increase after a peripheral vestibular damage.

Exercises in Bed

Eye movements:
- Looking up and then down.
- Looking alternatively left and right.
- Convergence exercises.

Head movements:
- Bending alternatively forward and backward.
- Turning alternatively to left and then right.

Exercises in Sitting Position

- Shrugging and rotating shoulders.
- Bending forward and picking up objects.
- Turning head and trunk alternately to the left and right.

Exercises in Standing Position

- Changing from sitting to standing, initially with eyes open and then with the eyes shut.
- Throwing a small ping-pong ball in an arc from hand to hand and following it with the eyes.
- Throwing a small ball from hand to hand under the knee.

Exercises while Walking
- Throwing and catching the ball while walking.
- Walking up and down a flight of stairs.
- Walking around in the room with eyes open and closed.
- Playing any game involving bending, stretching and aiming with the ball.

Surgical Treatment

There are specific conditions where surgical intervention may be needed such as a perilymph fistula or a superior semicircular canal dehiscence. Surgery can be considered for Ménière's disease and BPPV if medical or conventional management fails.

Surgical Options in Ménière's Disease
- *Endolymphatic sac surgery:* It has a 70–90% success rate and preserves hearing. It is reserved for patients who fail medical and aminoglycoside therapy.
- *Vestibular nerve section:* It has about 90% success rate. The vestibular nerve can be approached via the retrosigmoid or middle fossa route. It has risk of cerebrospinal fluid leak, facial palsy and hearing loss.
- *Labyrinthectomy:* It has a success rate around 95%. It can be done via a transcanal or transmastoid route. The aim of this procedure is to remove the membranous neuroepithelium from the vestibule and semicircular canals.
- *Intratympanic gentamycin:* It is a favored treatment in medically refractory patients. Success rate is around 90%. There is risk of hearing loss.
- *Intratympanic steroids:* Success rate is 50%. Intratympanic dexamethasone avoids the systemic complications of steroids. It may be considered for those with severe Ménière's disease in pregnancy.

Surgical Options in BPPV

Surgery for BPPV is done for intractable cases not responding to particle repositioning procedures or vestibular rehabilitation.

- *Singular neurectomy (Posterior ampullary nerve section):* Success rate is about 97%. There is risk of hearing loss.
- *Posterior semicircular canal occlusion:* Complete resolutions of symptoms in all patients have been reported. There is a risk of transient mild hearing loss.

SUMMARY

- The treatment of balance disorders must be definite and oriented to the etiology and pathogenesis of the condition.
- Pharmacotherapy, physiotherapy, psychotherapy or rarely surgery can be used for the management of balance disorders.
- The important medications useful in the treatment of balance disorders include anticholinergics, antihistamines, benzodiazepines, calcium-channel antagonists and dopamine-receptor antagonists.
- Symptomatic therapy must be reserved for acute episodes.
- In both Ménière's disease and vestibular neuronitis, vestibular suppressants such as anticholinergics and benzodiazepines are useful.
- In Ménière's disease, salt restriction and diuretics are used as a prophylaxis for flare-ups.
- Drug treatments are not recommended for benign paroxysmal positional vertigo and bilateral vestibular paresis, but physical therapy can be very useful in both.
- Prophylactic agents such as calcium-channel antagonists, tricyclic antidepressants and β-blockers are the mainstay of treatment for migraine-associated vertigo.
- Benzodiazepines are the most useful agents when psychogenic vertigo occurs in association with anxiety or agoraphobia.
- Vestibular rehabilitation therapy is generally recommended to improve quality of life.

Tips to Prevents Fall of Vertigo Patients in Old Age

- Always grab on to the hand-railing while climbing staircase.
- Install grab bar in bathrooms.
- Remember to mop-up wet and slippery areas.
- Ensure light switch and water are in easy reach during night.
- Preferable use of a three pronged walking stick for support.
- Avoid clutter on the floor, remember to tuck the edge of the carpet with a tape.

Vestibular Rehabilitation Exercises

Vestibular compensation occurs naturally in most patients, but not in all patients. In some patients, an incomplete compensation occurs. Incomplete or total failure of vestibular compensation is very distressing for the patient, since it leads to persistent instability and severely incapacitates the patient. These patients are very challenging. They can be rehabilitated properly.

Vestibular rehabilitation refers to a structured program of treatment aimed at expediting and enhancing vestibular compensation and rendering the dizzy patient asymptomatic. This is usually helpful for chronic vestibular symptoms due to unilateral labyrinthine pathology.

Usually, vestibular rehabilitation exercises are used for chronic or uncompensated vestibular disorders. However, its early use and benefit in managing acute peripheral vestibular disorders is increasingly recognized.

MECHANISMS

- *Habituation/adaptive responses:* It allow central nervous system to adjust changes in labyrinthine signals, e.g. ballet dancers and acrobats.
- *Sensory substitution:* It rely more on visual or proprioceptive input.

CAWTHRONE-COOKSEY EXERCISES

These exercises are a set of head, body and eye movement exercises for enhancing vestibular compensation in a patient of peripheral vestibular lesion. Patients recovered more rapidly using these techniques. These exercises can be broadly divided into three groups: Adaptation exercises, habituation exercises and compensation exercises.

- *Adaptation exercises:* Gaze stabilization exercises. It helps the patient with peripheral vestibular disorder to adopt the changed vestibular scenario by retraining the vestibulo-ocular reflex to stabilize images of moving objects in the fovea.
- *Habituation exercises:* It helps patients of peripheral vestibular disorder by conditioning the brain through repeated exposure of the balance system to erroneous or mismatched sensory input. For example, head (up and down), head (side to side), etc.
- *Compensation exercises:* The compensation or substitution exercises help the patient to enhance the visual and proprioceptive inputs so that the deficit of vestibular input is counterbalanced.

EYE EXERCISES

The eye movements as seen below enhance the adaptation as well as compensation. It helps the patient to enhance the visual and proprioceptive inputs so that the deficit of vestibular input is counterbalanced.

- Looking up and down **(Fig. 8.1)**.
- Looking alternatively left and right **(Fig. 8.2)**.
- Convergence exercises **(Fig. 8.3)**.

Vestibular Rehabilitation Exercises

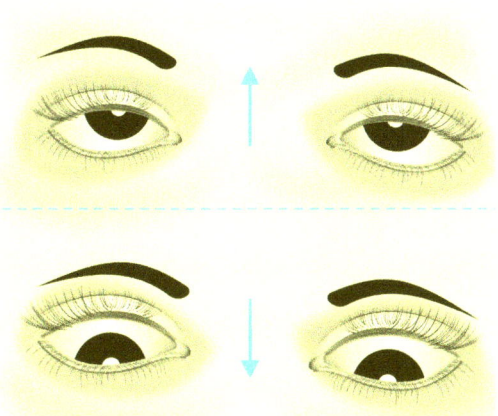

Fig. 8.1 Looking up and down

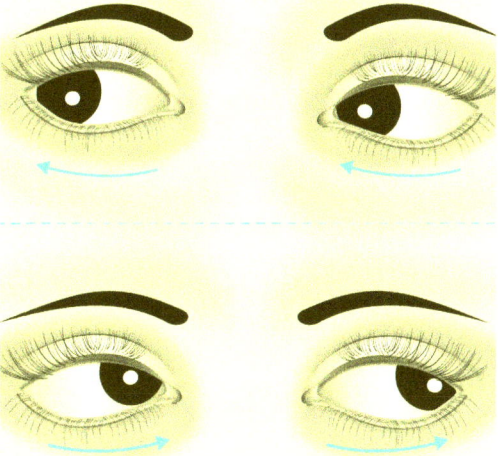

Fig. 8.2 Looking alternatively left and right

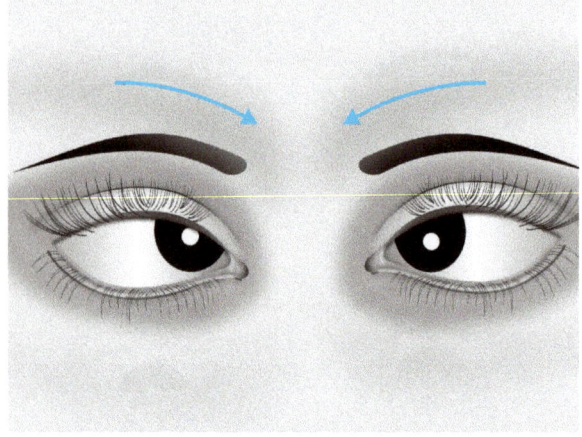

Fig. 8.3 Convergence exercises

HEAD AND NECK EXERCISES

This is habituation exercises. It helps the patients of peripheral vestibular disorder by conditioning the brain through repeated exposure of the balance system to erroneous or mismatched sensory inputs. These mismatched sensory inputs induce small tolerable spells of vertigo to which brain gets used to, so that minor vertiginous sensations are not bothersome to the patient. The patient carries out these exercises sitting up on the bed, or if one is stable enough, then sitting on a stool.

- Bending alternatively forward and backward (**Fig. 8.4**).
- Turning alternatively to left and then right (**Fig. 8.5**).

Exercises in Sitting Position

- Shrugging and rotating shoulders (**Fig. 8.6**).
- Bending forward and picking up objects from the floor (**Fig. 8.7**).
- Turning head and trunk alternatively to left and right (**Fig. 8.8**).

Vestibular Rehabilitation Exercises

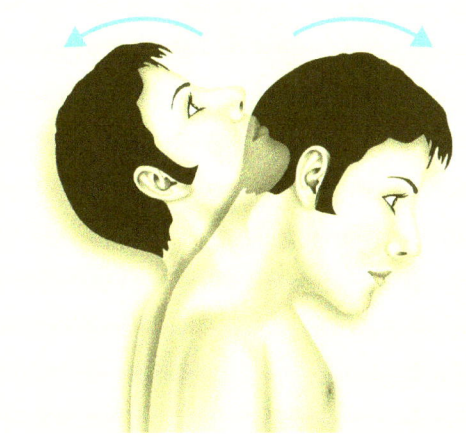

Fig. 8.4 Bending head forward and backward

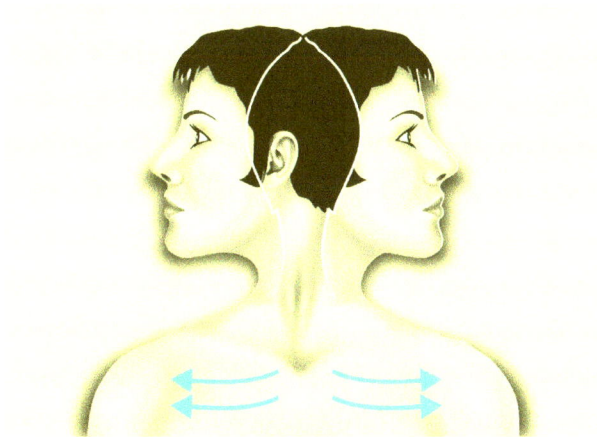

Fig. 8.5 Turning head to left and then right

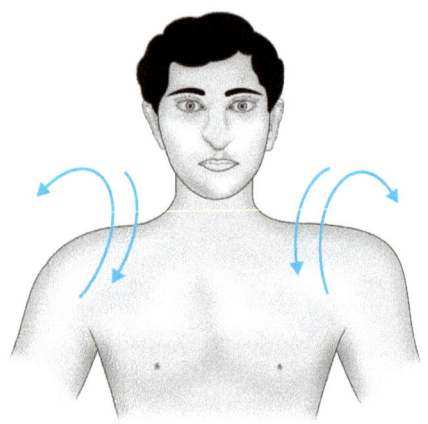

Fig. 8.6 Shrugging and rotating shoulders

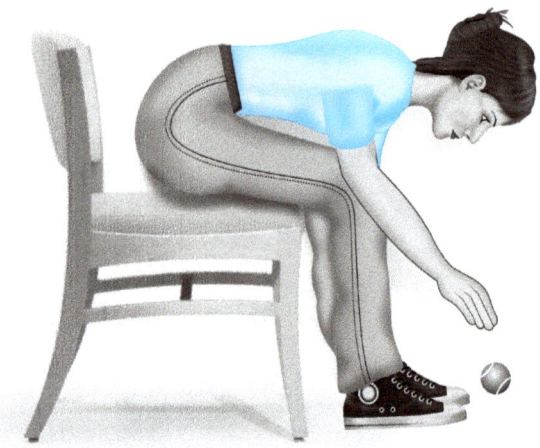

Fig. 8.7 Bending forward and picking up objects from the floor

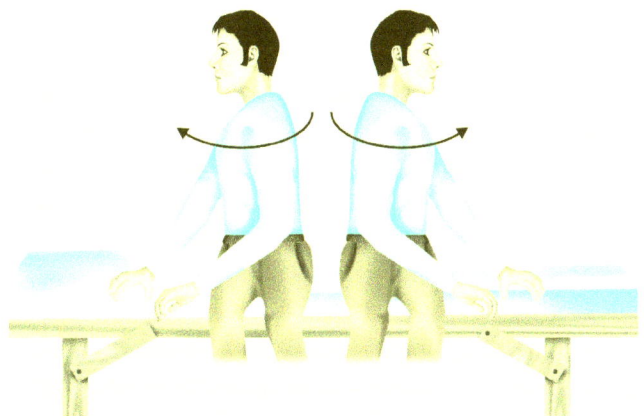

Fig. 8.8 Turning the head alternatively to left and right

Exercises in Standing Position

- Changing from sitting to standing, initially with eyes open and then with eyes shut repeatedly for 15 minutes (**Fig. 8.9**).
- Throwing a small ball is an arc from hand to hand and following the moving ball with eyes (**Fig. 8.10**).
  This is a gaze stabilization exercises which expedite adaptation. It helps the patient with peripheral vestibular disorder to adapt the changed vestibular scenario by retaining the vestibulo-ocular reflex to stabilize images of moving objects in the fovea. In this exercises, the movement of small rubber ball that the patient throws from one hand to the other repeatedly over the head. By this exercises, the extra-ocular muscles are retained to move the eyes in such a fashion that the eyes remain focused on the moving ball. In vestibular malfunction, images of moving objects can be kept fixed in the fovea by accurate and coordinated movements of the eyes.
- Throwing a small ball from hand to hand under the knee (**Fig. 8.11**).

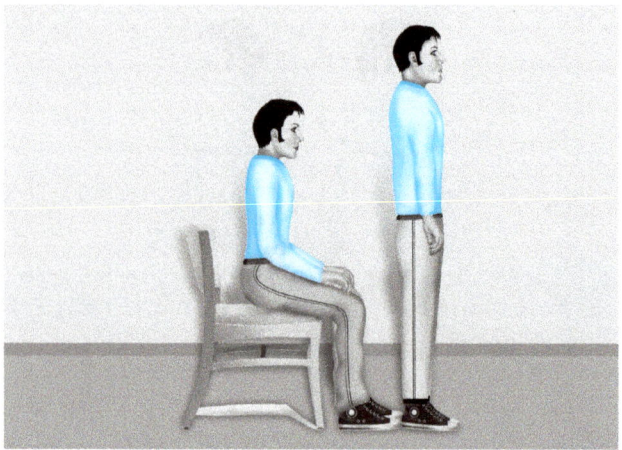

Fig. 8.9 Changing from sitting to standing position

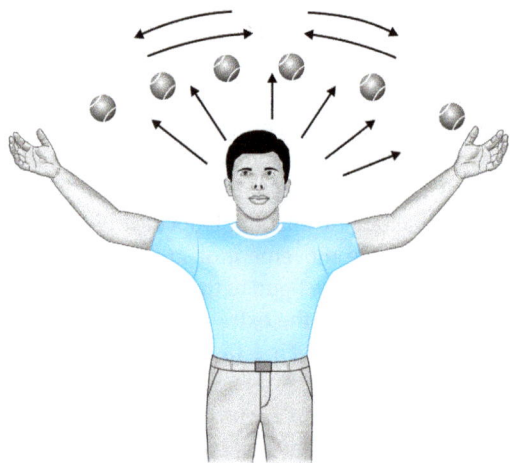

Fig. 8.10 Throwing a ball in an arc from hand to hand

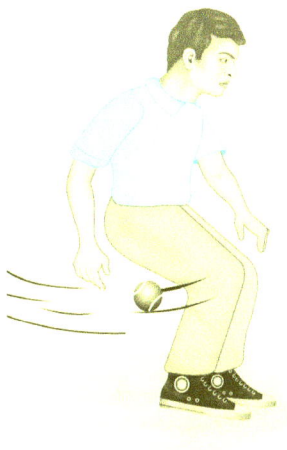

Fig. 8.11 Throwing a ball under the knee

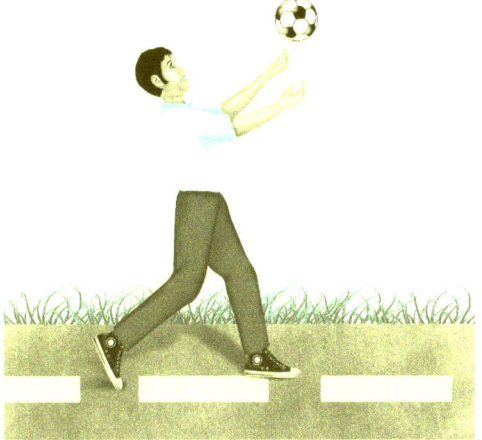

Fig. 8.12 Throwing and catching the ball

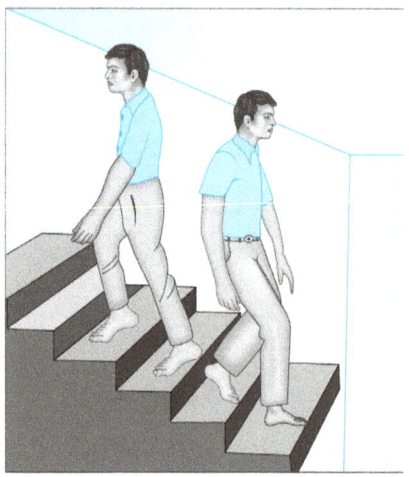

Fig. 8.13 Walking over stairs

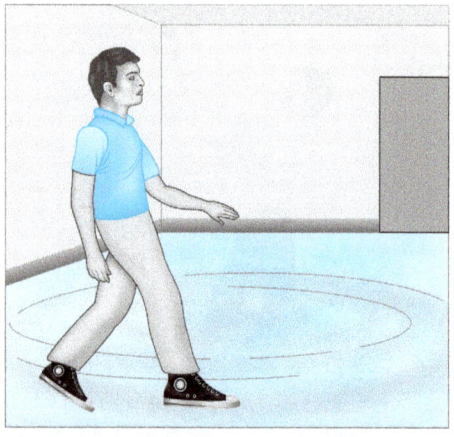

Fig. 8.14 Walking around inside the room with eye closed and open

Vestibular Rehabilitation Exercises

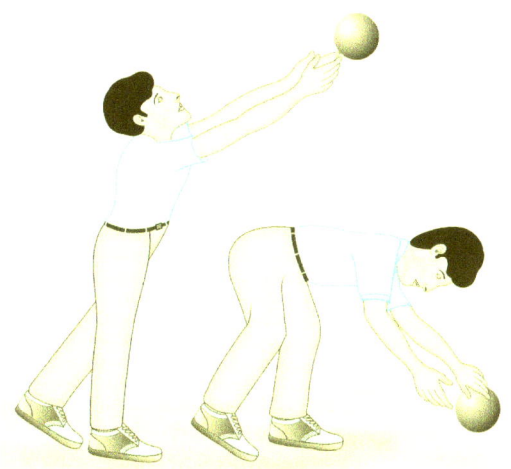

Fig. 8.15 Game for bending and stretching

Exercises while Walking

- Throwing and catching the ball while walking **(Fig. 8.12)**.
- Walking up and down a flight of stairs **(Fig. 8.13)**.
  Walking up and down a flight of stairs sensitizes the proprioceptive system and retains the balance system to rely more on proprioceptive rather than defective vestibular input.
- Walking around in the room with eyes closed and open **(Fig. 8.14)**.
- Playing any game involving bending, stretching and aiming with the ball **(Fig. 8.15)**.

CHAPTER 9

Important Clinical Conditions of Vertigo

MÉNIÈRE'S DISEASE

- Ménière's disease typically has a triad of attacks of vertigo, fluctuating tinnitus, fluctuating sensorineural hearing loss and fullness in the ear (**Table 9.1**).
- The attack of vertigo typically lasting from 1/2 to 24 hours and many occur per week or separated by years.
- The course is unpredictable but generally progressive and it often becomes bilateral.
- Ménière's disease may be wrongly diagnosed in patients with mild tinnitus or deafness due to other causes.
- One should be careful not to miss BPPV or migraine, unless the pattern of vertigo, hearing loss and tinnitus is typical.

Objective of Treatment of Ménière's Disease

- To treat acute attack.
- To prevent further attacks.

Table 9.1 Ménière's triad	
Hearing loss	Fluctuants, worsens during vertigo spells and is associated with aural fullness
Tinnitus	Fluctuates, can have a roaring quality and is louder during vertigo spells
Vertigo	Is usually hours in duration, severe, and associated with vomiting

Important Clinical Conditions of Vertigo

- To prevent and/or preserve hearing and vestibular function.
- To prevent development of bilateral Ménière's disease.

Management Protocol in Ménière's Disease

If the practitioner can reach a very conclusive diagnosis from the history, clinical examination, audiometry and vestibulometry, a CT scan or MRI is not needed. But sometimes these tests become necessary not only to exclude an intracranial pathology but also to allay the fear of a serious life-threatening problem in the patient's mind.

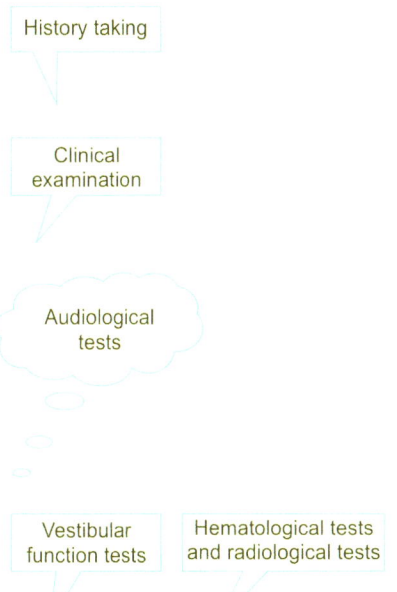

Treatment

Acute Attack

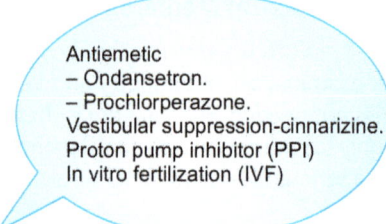

Antiemetic
– Ondansetron.
– Prochlorperazone.
Vestibular suppression-cinnarizine.
Proton pump inhibitor (PPI)
In vitro fertilization (IVF)

Remission

```
Diet control
   ↓
Vasodilators: Betahistine
   ↓
Diuretics: Acetazolamide, triametrene
   ↓
Intratympanic ototoxic injection
```

Surgery

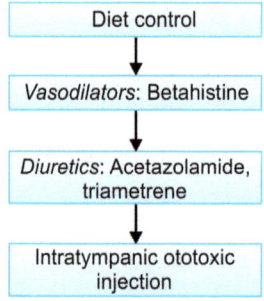

- Endolymphatic sac surgery.
- Vestibular neurectomy.
- Labyrinthectomy

Important Clinical Conditions of Vertigo

BENIGN PAROXYSMAL POSITIONAL VERTIGO (BPPV)

- It is the most common cause of vertigo.
- The patient is usually extremely scared and disabled by the vertigo and unsteadiness.
- This condition is often wrongly blamed on cervical spondylosis (which is an extremely common X-ray finding in people above age 30 or 40 years), low or high blood pressure, low blood sugar, less blood supply to the brain, etc.
- The diagnosis of BPPV is very easy and it is one condition which can probably be fairly confidently diagnosed on the phone. The patient describes brief attacks lasting less than a minute of positional vertigo, triggered by rolling over in bed, looking up or down or turning head to one side.
- The most common test used for BPPV diagnosis is the Dix-Hallpike maneuver, which can be done by the ENT specialist in his office. First, the patient seats in the stretcher. The patient's head should be turned 45° towards the side to be tested. The patient lays and has the head hyperextended about 20°. If the maneuver is positive, the patient relates vertigo and the examiner is able to observe the typical nystagmus.

VESTIBULAR NEURONITIS

- The vestibular neuronitis, also called epidemic vertigo.
- It is characterized by violent and sudden vertigo followed by nauseas and vomiting.
- It is the second most common peripheral cause of vestibular vertigo.

Clinical Presentations

- Severe and longstanding sudden vertigo lasting for days.
- No hearing loss.

- Occuring predominantly in the middle age, affecting both genders equally.
- Association with recent or recurrent respiratory infection of upper airways.
- Significant reduction or absence of response to the thermal tests on the affected side.
- Absence of neurological symptoms or findings.
- Since the majority of the patients present a satisfactory recovery, the initial treatment is solely symptomatic, involving rest, antiemetics and hydration. Vestibular depressors should be used only in the acute phase, with gradual withdrawal in days or weeks, based on the hypothesis that the continuous and lingering use of these medications can hinder the central vestibular compensation.

PERILYMPH FISTULA

- A perilymph fistula is an abnormal connection between the middle ear and inner ear, usually after disruption of the lining membranes of the labyrinth or the oval or round window.
- Head trauma, rapid or profound changes in intracranial or atmospheric pressure (scuba diving, air travel), violent sneezing, coughing or lifting are the most common causes of fistula.
- Otologic surgery, cholesteatoma and congenital dehiscence of the labyrinthine bone can also cause perilymph fistula.
- Patients typically report episodes of vertigo, dizziness, nausea and vomiting, which often worsen with activity or Valsalva maneuvers.
- Loud noises or the use of one's own voice can also cause vertigo (Tullio's phenomenon).
- Hearing loss and tinnitus are mostly associated with the vestibular symptoms.

Important Clinical Conditions of Vertigo

- During a fistula test, which entails observing eye movements while changing the air pressure in the external auditory canal, nystagmus can be observed.
- CT scans can show bony dehiscences of the semicircular canals or indirect signs of perilymph fistula, such as pneumolabyrinth or middle ear effusions.
- Treatment of perilymph fistulas usually consists of patching of the fistula with a soft tissue graft and fibrin glue. In rare cases, where sensorineural hearing loss is not associated with the vestibular symptoms, conservative approaches with restriction of physical activity and avoidance of pressure changes can be helpful.
- *Tullio's phenomenon or Hennebert's sign:* They are present in patients with labyrinthine fistula and perilymphatic fistula.

SUPERIOR SEMICIRCULAR CANAL DEHISCENCE

- Superior canal dehiscence is absence of the bony roof of the superior semicircular canal.
- Superior semicircular canal dehiscence differs from a perilymph fistula in that the former there is no direct communication with an air-filled cavity while in the latter, there is a tear in the membrane which communicates directly with an air-filled cavity.
- The symptoms of this condition and perilymph fistula are triggered by ear pressure, sound and increase in intrathoracic pressure, but less severe in dehiscence.
- The superior canal dehiscence can be congenital, due to trauma, surgery or cholesteatoma.
- Patient of this condition complains unsteadiness with activity and relieved with rest.
- They have conductive deafness.
- They have Valsalva-induced dizziness—worsening of symptoms with coughing, sneezing and blowing of nose.

- *Tullio's phenomenon is positive:* Dizziness induced by loud sounds. It also occurs in Ménière's disease and perilymph fistula.
- *Autophony:* Patient find that their voice sounds louder than normal. In the patulous Eustachian tube, the eardrum will show movement with respiration.
- Hennebert's sign is positive.
- Fistula test is positive. A negative test does not exclude the condition.
- High resolution CT scans of the temporal bone shows the defect of superior semicircular canal.
- *Treatment:*
  Conservative: Lifestyle modification with avoidance of aggravating factors
  Surgery: Plugging of the superior semicircular canal.

LABYRINTHITIS

- Labyrinthitis is an infection of the entire labyrinth or the entire 8th nerve (vestibulocochlear).
- It can be bacterial or viral in origin.
- Clinical features are similar to vestibular neuritis with the additional symptoms of hearing loss and tinnitus.
- Bacterial labyrinthitis need appropriate antibiotics, depending on the source of infection (e.g. meningitis, chronic suppurative otitis media) and surgical management of the infective foci, if necessary.
- Labyrinthine sedatives given for symptomatic treatment.

ACOUSTIC NEUROMA

- Acoustic neuromas are slow growing tumors (1 mm/year).
- Patients with an acoustic neuroma (vestibular schwannoma) present with hearing loss, tinnitus and imbalance or unsteadiness. They do not present true vertigo.

Important Clinical Conditions of Vertigo

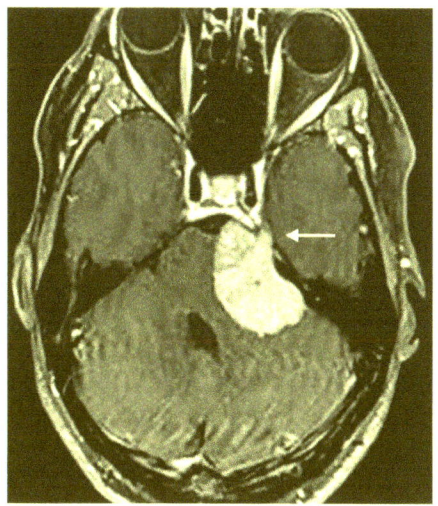

Fig. 9.1 MRI brain showing acoustic neuroma

- There is loss of ipsilateral corneal reflex from involvement of the trigeminal nerve.
- MRI with gadolinium contrast is the gold standard for diagnosis of acoustic neuroma **(Fig. 9.1)**.
- Surgical removal of tumor is the treatment of choice.

BILATERAL VESTIBULOPATHY

- There is loss of afferent vestibular input from the labyrinth.
- This disorder is characterized by postural imbalance and oscillopsia during head movements.
- Most cases are idiopathic or caused by aminoglycoside toxicity.
- 'Catch-up' saccades are seen following head impulses in all directions.
- Vestibular rehabilitation helps to improve postural stability.

AUTOIMMUNE LABYRINTHITIS

- The autoimmune dysfunction of the inner ear may occur as part of systemic lupus erythematosus (SLE), polyarteritis nodosa, etc.
- It usually affects middle-aged females and is commonly bilateral; though it may start unilaterally.
- Gradually increasing sensorineural deafness with vertiginous symptoms occasionally having spells of acute exacerbation is the usual clinical picture.
- Audiovestibular investigations show evidence of cochlear type of sensorineural deafness usually with bilateral canal paresis.
- *Blood tests:* Erythrocyte sedimentation rate (ESR), rheumatoid factor, immunoglobulins, antinuclear antibodies, etc.
- Cogan's syndrome is one of the localized varieties of autoimmune inner ear disorder and consists of a combination of interstitial keratitis and inner ear disorder—sometimes accompanied with aortitis.
- Steroids are the mainstay of treatment.

CENTRAL CAUSES OF VERTIGO

- Central vertigo is usually associated with severe vertigo with neurologic signs and less prominent movement illusion.
- The presence of pure vertical and multidirectional nystagmus with no optical fixation suppression is usually indicative of central cause of vertigo.
- Epidemiologic studies demonstrated that central causes comprise approximately 25% of vertigo experienced in patients.
- Central vertigo requiring emergency intervention are cerebellar infarction or hemorrhage, basilar artery occlusion, vertebral artery dissection and a tumor of the posterior cranial fossa.

Migrainous Vertigo

- It is a disorder characterized by episodic headache associated with vertigo.
- Patients have recurrent attacks of spontaneous or positional vertigo.
- There may or may not be an associated headache always.
- Some patients have vertigo as their migrainous aura and then go on to develop a typical hemicranial headache. Other patients have vertigo that begins with the headache or appears later in the headache phase, while most have attacks of vertigo without any associated headache.
- Some patients have photobhobia, phonophobia or visual auras in association with their vertigo attacks.
- This patient usually responds well to lifestyle changes, migraine treatment and prophylaxis.

Wallenberg's Syndrome

- It is also known as lateral medullary infarction.
- It is usually caused by an occlusion of the ipsilateral vertebral artery that supplies the posteroinferior cerebellar artery, leading to acute onset of vertigo.
- The neurologic deficits include abnormal eye movements, ipsilateral Horner's syndrome, ipsilateral limb ataxia and loss of pain/temperature sensation on ipsilateral face and contralateral trunk.

Cerebellar Infarction and Hemorrhage

- It mainly affects older patients and usually produces sudden vertigo associated with nausea and vomiting.
- Limb ataxia and impaired gait are suggestive of cerebellar lesion.

Multiple Sclerosis

- It has been reported that vertigo occurs in 20–25% of the multiple sclerosis patients.
- Vertigo usually lasts days to weeks and symptoms may resemble vestibular neuronitis.
- Depending on the location of the demyelinating plaques, the associated findings may vary.
- Dysfunction of adjacent cranial nerves (facial numbness, diplopia) or cerebellar signs (severe vertigo) may be present.

Brainstem Ischemia

- Vertebrobasillar transient ischemic attacks of the brainstem are characterized by episodic vertigo lasting minutes to hours.
- There are concurrent neurological symptoms such as diplopia, dysarthria and ataxia.

Posterior Fossa Tumors

- Intrinsic tumors, such as cerebellar tumors, may result in a progressive onset of headache, postural imbalance and positional vertigo.
- Extrinsic tumors, such as vestibular schwannomas, may result in a progressive onset of unilateral hearing loss and tinnitus.
- MRI with gadolinium contrast is useful for diagnosis.
- Treatment depends on the size, location and type of tumor present.

Vertebrobasilar Insufficiency (VBI)

- It is also known as transient ischemic attack (TIA) of the vertebrobasilar system.
- Among elderly patients, VBI is a common cause of vertigo.

- Thromboembolism and hemodynamic compromises are the major two pathological mechanisms that lead to vertebrobasilar insufficiency.
- Vertebrobasilar insufficiency is more likely in patients with history of stroke, concomitant coronary or peripheral artery disease, hyperlipidemia, hypertension, diabetes mellitus, tobacco use, strong family history of stroke or recent neck trauma.
- Vertigo is the most frequent and sometimes the only symptom in VBI. Typically, VBI-associated vertigo occurs in attacks, depends on position, and is frequently associated with nystagmus, nausea, vomiting and severe imbalance. Concomitant symptoms include blurred vision, blackouts, drop attacks or headache.
- Vertigo associated with VBI typically lasts minutes.
- The management objective in VBI is to improve impaired circulation and to restore normal perfusion of compromised areas. Patients who present with a TIA or stroke due to atherosclerosis require aggressive medical management with an antiplatelet agent, anticoagulant lowering of their blood pressure to <130/80 mm Hg, low density lipoprotein (LDL) cholesterol to <70 mg/dL, and adequate control of their blood sugar, in addition lifestyle changes (diet, exercises and tobacco cessation).
- Vascular insufficiency/cerebral ischemia leading to dizziness and unsteadiness apparently responds to cinnarizine, a calcium channel blocker. It helps by improving the microcirculation in cerebral tissue/inner ear.

MOTION SICKNESS

Motion sickness or kinetosis is a syndrome characterized by nausea, vomiting, pallor, dizziness and cold with sweating which is induced when an individual is exposed to certain types of real or apparent motion stimuli. Motion sickness is not a pathological but is the normal response of an individual, with an intact vestibular system, to motion stimuli with which he is unfamiliar and to which he is unadapted.

Clinical Features

- Earliest symptom is sensation of epigastric discomfort-stomach awareness.
- Nausea, pallor and sweating.
- Feeling bodily warmth and the individual seeks cool air to obtain relief.
- Dizziness and headache.
- Vomiting and retching.
- After vomiting there is temporary relief followed by deterioration of condition.
- Time course of adaptation is 2 to 4 hours.

Etiology

- Vestibular overstimulation.
- Presence of sensory information about bodily motion which is at variance with inputs that, the central nervous system would expect to receive—Neural mismatch.

Behavioral Measures

- Minimize unnecessary head movements and keep the body restraint.
- Occupy a position abroad the ship or aircraft close to its center of gravity in order to minimize the intensity of motion stimuli.
- Maintain a position where there is a good forward view.
- If there is deprived visual field, close the eyes to reduce the visual-vestibular conflict.
- Be involved in a task which occupies the mind.

Important Clinical Conditions of Vertigo

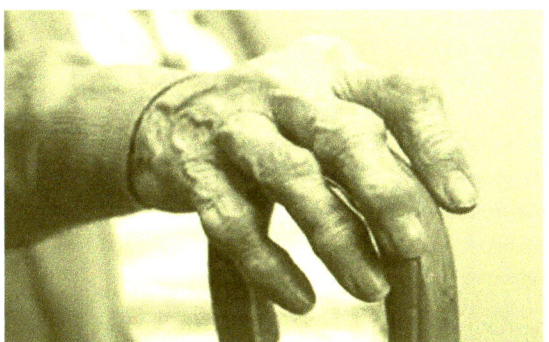

Fig. 9.2 Elderly person suffering with imbalance

Medical Measures

- Hyoscine hydrobromide 0. 3–0.6 mg acts in 30–60 minutes and provides protection for 4 hours.
- Promethazine hydrochloride 25 mg.
- Meclazine HCl 50 mg.
- Cyclizine HCl 50 mg.
- Cinnarizine 25 mg.

Transdermal therapeutic hyoscine adhesive patch kept behind ears gives a loading dose of 200 micrograms and controlled release at 10 micrograms/hour for up to 48 hours.

Vertigo in Elderly Person (Fig. 9.2)

Elderly people can have vertigo due to all of the causes that middle aged patients and even younger can have vertigo. The difference is that elderly patients may be associated with other systemic problems which will enhance their vertigo. Systemic problems like visual or neurological or orthopedic or gastrointestinal can confound the dizziness of the elderly patients. So when approaching for the treatment of vertigo in elderly, both true vertigo and systemic problems are properly managed.

CHAPTER 10

Approach to Vertigo by General Practitioner

General practitioners (GP) are the first line physicians in the vertigo management. Patients with giddiness or imbalance always seek immediate medical help from his/her nearest doctor (GP). General practitioner should have basic knowledge in the diagnosis and management of vertigo so that patients will immediate relief. They should also know which patients should be referred immediately to the consultants.

Basic information regarding vertigo should be known to GP.

- **Episodic dizziness**
  - Benign paroxysmal positional vertigo (BPPV): Manage at Primary care by doing Epley's maneuver. If fails—refer to ENT specialist.
  - Postural hypotension or migraine—refer to physician.
  - Associated otologic symptoms/signs—ENT referral.
- **Acute dizziness**
  - Suspected myocardial infarction/neurological findings/ Unsure—Refer to tertiary center.
  - Unstable patient or dehydrated patient—hospital admission.
  - Stable patient or gastrointestinal infection—manage at primary care.
- **Chronic/persistent dizziness**
  - Drugs/anemia—manage at primary care.
  - Associated ear findings—refer to ENT.
  - Neurological findings/unsure—physician referral.

DIAGNOSIS OF OTOLOGIC VERTIGO

- **Vertigo (Minutes to hours)**
  - Hearing loss, tinnitus, ear pressure, usually spontaneous, horizontal nystagmus—Ménière's disease.
- **Vertigo (Seconds)**
  - No auditory symptoms, triggered by head position, crystals in the posterior semicircular canal, rotatory nystagmus—benign paroxysmal positional vertigo.
- **Vertigo (Days to weeks)**
  - No auditory symptoms, commonly after upper respiratory infection, viral infection of vestibular nerve, horizontal nystagmus—vestibular neuronitis/viral labyrinthitis.
- **Vertigo (Minutes to hours)**
  - No auditory symptoms, usually spontaneous, recurrent deafferentation of vestibular nerve, horizontal nystagmus—recurrent vestibulopathy.

CONDITIONS REQUIRING URGENT REFERRAL TO BALANCE SPECIALIST

- Presence of auditory symptoms (hearing loss, tinnitus, pressure or aural fullness, particularly, if asymmetrical).
- Nystagmus has central features.
- Spontaneous and persists after 48 hours.
- Signs of suppurative otitis media.
- Auditory or vestibular symptoms are triggered by pressure changes (barotraumas or Valsalva maneuver), suggestive of perilymph fistula.
- Progressive unsteadiness or falls.
- Cardiovascular symptoms (chest pain, dyspnea, syncope, etc.).

SIMPLIFIED APPROACH TO GET A DIAGNOSIS

If patient complaints with vertigo or dizziness.

True Vertigo (Hallucination of Rotation or Imbalance Felt within the Head)

If there are features of true vertigo: Consider following:
- Is there evidence of middle ear disease (discharge, perforation, cholesteatoma, mastoiditis)?
  – Infection may spread to affect labyrinth. Requires full otological assessment.
  – Refer to otologist.
- Is patient receiving any vestibulotoxic drugs (aminoglycosides, anticonvulsants, furosemide, ethacrynic acid, anti-inflammatories, salicylates, quinine)?
  – Damage may be transient (e.g. phenytoin) or permanent (e.g. gentamicin).
  – Stop or reduce.
- Are there any focal neurological signs?
  – Yes.
  – Cranial nerve palsies, cerebellar or long tract damage, visual disturbance.
  – Consider: In young patients multiple sclerosis, migraine, vasculitis; in older patients vertebrobasilar disease, neoplasia.
  – Refer for neurological assessment.
- Do patients have tinnitus or constitutional upset, e.g. nausea, vomiting, sweating?
  – Yes.
  – Is hearing impaired.
    - Yes.
    - Sensorineural deafness.
  – Are symptoms recurrent?
  – Ménière's disease.
  – Treatment: Bed rest and give drugs such as cinnarizine, prochlorperazine and surgery for severe Ménière's disease.

- Are there focal neurological signs? With tinnitus and unilateral sensorineural hearing loss
  - Yes.
  - Progressive.
  - Yes.
  - Consider cerebellopontine angle tumor, especially acoustic neuroma.
  - Refer to neurosurgeon for further management.
- Is vertigo associated with a particular head position?
  - Yes.
  - Benign positional vertigo confirmed by positional test.
  - Reassure of benign nature and limited duration. Avoidance or provocative positions and do Epley maneuver.
- Is there a history of head injury?
  - Yes.
  - Vertigo may be associated with closed injury, with or without skull fracture, and out of proportion with severity of trauma.
  - Prognosis good but recovery may be protracted.
  - Supportive treatment.
- Is vertigo associated with motion, e.g. driving, sea travel?
  - Yes.
  - Motion sickness.
  - Treatment: Avoidance of motion, antihistamines.

Dizziness (Not True vertigo)

- *Symptoms of imbalance felt in the legs:* Look for evidence of cerebellar disease, proprioceptive damage, muscular weakness
  - Consult neurologist.
- *Do symptoms suggest postural hypotension:* Measure erect and supine blood pressure?
  - Postural hypotension.

- Consider drugs, alcohol, diabetes, anemia, Addison's disease, autonomic neuropathy.
- If BP is raised
  - Investigate and treat as appropriate.
- Are there any cardiac signs?
  - Yes.
  - Like dysrhythmia, murmurs, cardiac failure, abnormal ECG.
  - Refer to cardiologist for treatment.
- Are there features suggestive of epilepsy?
  - Yes.
  - Symptoms may reflect: Aura or fits especially temporal lobe epilepsy, anticonvulsant toxicity.
  - EEG may be required and neurology consultation.
- Is there evidence of anemia or polycythemia?
  - Yes.
  - Check full blood count, blood film.
  - Investigate further as appropriate.
- Do symptoms suggest hypoglycemia?
  - Yes.
  - Is patient taking insulin or sulfonylureas?
    - Yes.
  - Is patient: Taking the correct dose? Receiving insufficient food? Taking inappropriate exercise? Is control too tight?
  - Modify treatment and improve patient education.
- *Symptoms of hypoglycemia:*
  - Patient is not taking insulin/sulfonylureas.
  - *Consider:* Reactive hypoglycemia, e.g. postgastrectomy, Addisson's disease, hypopituitarism, insulinoma.
  - Investigate and treat as appropriate.
- Are symptoms related to neck movements?
  - Yes.
  - This may reflect cervical spondylosis, carotid sinus hypersensitivity (rare).
  - If association is definite, collar may help.

- Are there features of psychiatric disturbance?
    - Yes.
    - Anxiety disorders or panic attack with hyperventilation are most common.
    - Are symptoms reproduced by voluntary overbreathing?
        - No.
    - *Consider:* Depression, psychosis, hypochondriasis.
    - Consult psychiatrist.
- If above symptoms are reproduced by voluntary overbreathing?
    - Hyperventilation confirmed.
    - *Treatment:* Controlled breathing training.

GUIDING FOR EVALUATION OF DIZZY PATIENTS (FLOW CHART 10.1)

History

- *Description:*
    - *Vertigo:* Sensation of motion or spinning.
    - *Presyncope:* Blacking out or loss of consciousness.
    - *Disequilibrium:* Loss of balance or woobly.
    - Lightheadedness.
- *Duration:*
    - Seconds-minutes.
    - Hours.
    - Days.
- *Onset:*
    - Sudden.
    - Chronic.
- *Frequency:*
    - Acute.
    - Episodic.
    - Persistent.

Flow chart 10.1 Guide for vertigo practice by general practitioner

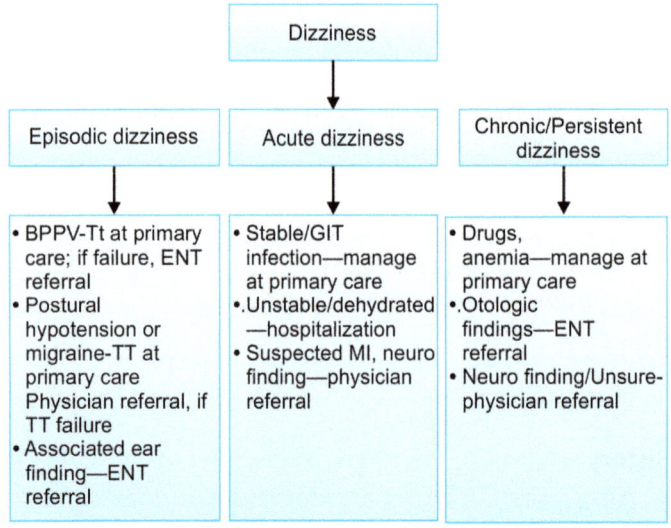

- *Aggravating factors:*
  - Position.
  - Coughing.
  - Loud sounds.
  - Stress, fatigue, hunger, emotional upset and menses.
- *Associated symptoms:*
  - *Otologic symptoms:* Hearing loss, tinnitus, ear fullness or pain or ear discharge.
  - *Neurological symptoms:* Headache, aura, visual disturbance, numbness, weakness, speech and swallowing difficulties.
- *Past medical history:*
  - Cardiovascular disease.
  - Endocrine and metabolic disease.
  - Migraine.
  - Psychiatric illness.

- *Drug history:*
  - *Ototoxic drugs:* Antimlarial, antituberculous, topical antibiotic eardrops, aminoglycosides and chemotherapeutic drugs.
  - Antihypertensives.
  - Antiepileptics.
  - Sedatives and drugs acting on the central nervous system.

Examinations

General Examination

- Pallor.
- Blood pressure.
- Pulse.
- Temperature.
- Postural hypotension.

ENT Examination

- Otoscopy.
- Rinne'e and Weber's test.

Neurologic Examination

- *Cranial nerve examinations:* Normal/abnormal.
- *Upper and lower limb examination:* Tone, power, sensation, reflexes.

Neurotologic Examination

- Spontaneous and gaze-evoked nystagmus.
- *Oculomotor tests:* Fixation, smooth pursuit, saccades, convergence—positive in central lesions.
- *Special vestibular tests (VOR):* Head shake test, Halmagyl, VOR suppression, oscillopsia.

- *Tests for vestibulospinal tract:* Gait, Romberg's test.
- *Cerebellar test:* Past pointing/Dysdiadochokinesia.
- *Tests for mechanical disorders of the semicircular canals:* Dix-Hallpike test, fistula test, Valsalva. These are positive in peripheral lesions.
- *Tests for utricular dysfunction (otolith-ocular reflexes):* Skew deviation, Ocular tilt reaction, subjective visual vertical. These are seen in both peripheral and central lesions.

Investigations

- *Audiological test:*
  - Pure tone audiometry.
- *Hematolgical tests:*
  - Full blood count.
  - Fasting blood sugar.
  - Thyroid function test.
  - Venereal disease research laboratory (VDRL).
  - Cardiac enzymes.
  - Blood urea and serum electrolytes.
  - Autoimmune screening.
- *Cardiological test:*
  - Electrocardiogram (ECG).
- *Radiological tests:*
  - CT scan.
  - MRI.
- *Special vestibular tests:*
  - ENG/VNG.
  - Video head impulse test.
  - Vestibular evoked myogenic potentials (VEMP).
  - Caloric tests.
  - Electrocochleography.
  - Dynamic posturography.
  - Rotatory chair.

CHAPTER 11

Interesting Case Series

CASE 1: VESTIBULAR NEURONITIS

Case Presentation
A 60-year-old housewife presented with complaints of severe rotator, spinning sensation since one week. She had nausea and vomiting during the episodes. She had also instability on walking since one week. After taking by a general practitioner, she had an improvement in her symptoms. However, instability while walking persisted. She had no hearing loss or tinnitus.

Past History
- She is not diabetic and hypertensive.
- She was not taking any ototoxic medication before attack.
- She gave history of viral rhinitis about 15 days prior to presentation.

Clinical Examination
- Both tympanic membranes are normal.
- Tuning fork tests are normal.
- All cranial nerves, motor, sensory systems and reflexes are found to be normal.
- No cerebellar signs seen.
- Horizontal nystagmus of first degree beating to the left.

- *Unterberger's stepping test:* Abnormal deviation and rotation to the left.
- Gaze test, positional test and Dix-Hallpike test are normal.

Investigations

- Pure tone audiometry is within normal limit.
- Electronystagmography (ENG) done at the time of presentation showed spontaneous nystagmus to the left. Caloric test showed right-sided hypoactive responses to warm and cold water irrigation.

Diagnosis and Discussion

This is a typical case of vestibular neuronitis. Patient presents with severe rotator vertigo along with nausea and vomiting lasting for a week. There are no ear symptoms such as deafness, tinnitus, aural fullness, headache, diplopia or any sensory-motor loss. Classically, it is preceded by an attack of upper respiratory tract infection, yet in most cases (70%), this history may not be present. So, the absence of history of upper respiratory tract infection does not rule out vestibular neuritis.

Treatment

- The drug therapy for vestibular neuritis comprises of vestibular sedatives and antiemetics, primarily to provide symptomatic relief. The patient may be started with antivertigo drugs.
- The mainstay of therapy for long-term relief is early mobilization and vestibular rehabilitation exercises.

CASE 2: MÉNIÈRE'S DISEASE

Case Presentation

A 35-year-old man presented with recurrent attacks of giddiness for last 5 years. The attacks were infrequent initially, but over the last 1 year, the attacks have occurred at gradually shorter intervals. The attacks were accompanied by severe nausea, occasionally with vomiting, tinnitus and heaviness of the right ear. Each of the attacks lasted for 1 to 6 hours, but the patient's uneasiness and sense of instability persisted for about a day. In between two consecutive attacks, the patient was normal, but for last 6 months he experienced persistent heaviness in the right ear.

General ENT Examination

- General condition of patient is normal.
- Clinically ENT examination did not reveal any remarkable abnormality.
- No facial weakness was noted.
- Corneal reflex was normally bilateral.

Clinical Neurotological Examination

- Standing test and stepping test are normal.
- Positional test normal.
- No nystagmus obtained in headshaking test.

Investigations

- Pure tone audiometry test showed a mild-to-moderate degree of sensorineural deafness slightly more marked in the lower frequencies on the right side with normal hearing level on the left.
- Tone decay test was negative bilaterally.
- ABLB test showed complete recruitment.
- Glycerol test was positive.
- Electronystagmography (ENG) showed a hypoactive caloric response in right side with normal response on the left side.

Diagnosis

This typical case of Ménière's disease of the right side.

CASE 3: BENIGN PAROXYSMAL POSITIONAL VERTIGO (BPPV)

Case Presentation

A 50-year-old male presented with repeated attacks of occasional rotator vertigo with severe nausea but no vomiting. Each attack lasting for about 1 minute for 2 weeks. Symptoms induced on turning usually in bed but sometimes even while sitting. Several times, the symptoms were elicited when the patients tried to get up from bed. He has no deafness, tinnitus, aural fullness and muscular weakness.

Examinations

- Otoscopic examination—normal.
- Tuning fork test—normal.
- No cranial nerve palsy.
- No motor/sensory deficit.
- Plantar flexor and deep tendon reflex normal.
- No spontaneous nystagmus.
- Dix-Hallpike test showed definite rotatory left beating nystagmus (anticlockwise direction) in left lateral position of head. Nystagmus started after about 10 seconds and accompanied by severe vertigo and mild nausea. The nystagmus and vertigo subsided after about 30–40 seconds. Repeating the position reduced the vertigo significantly.
- Unterburger's stepping test, standing test and cerebellar tests were all normal.

Investigations

Pure tone audiometry—normal.

Diagnosis

This is classical case of left side BPPV.

CASE 4: MÉNIÈRE'S DISEASE

A 45-year-old man working as a clerk in a office presented with frequent attacks of severe giddiness with nausea and vomiting, each attack persisting for about 2 to 5 hours and on occasion, it continues for nearly day. The patient has been experiencing these attacks of giddiness for about 3 to 4 years. Initially, these attacks used to occur once every 2 to 3 months, but lately the frequency has been increased and now these attacks of giddiness occur 3 to 4 times a month. Now, he finds difficult to attend office, feels incapacitated, has become extremely depressed and frustrated, stays at home more than 10 days a month. Additionally, the patient has deafness and tinnitus in right ear, which has been there for the last 3 years so, but during the attacks of giddiness, the tinnitus increases, and there is also a definite sense of fullness and blockage of the right ear just prior to and during attack. Very often, he can predict an impending attack as the sense of blockage of the right ear and the increase of tinnitus usually starts as few hours before the onset of giddiness.

Clinical Diagnosis: Ménière's Disease

Explanations

The typical triad of vertigo-deafness-tinnitus accompanied by a sense of aural fullness and the episodic nature of the attack is by itself very typical of Ménière's disease. The patient is perfectly normal in between two successive attacks (except for deafness and mild tinnitus) proves the episodic nature of the disease, which is the very characteristic of Ménière's disease.

CASE-5: MIGRAINE-RELATED VERTIGO

A 40-year-old male executive reported with recurrent attacks of vertigo each attack persisting for 2 to 4 hours with no accompanying symptoms. There were no precipitating factors that the patient could recall on asking leading questions about any ear symptoms such as tinnitus, deafness or aural fullness, the patient categorically denied any related ear symptoms. The vertiginous attacks had been occurring once every 2–3 months for the last 2 years but for the last 3 months, it is much more frequent occurring once or twice every week.

Important History Noted
- Recurrent attacks of vertigo with no accompanying symptoms.
- No ear symptoms noted.
- Duration of each symptom is 2–4 hours.
- Patient state in between two attacks—Nothing specified.

Past History
- Patient had undergone angioplasty 5 years back for cardiac problems.
- He has a mild persistent pain in shoulder 2 years back diagnosed cervical spondylosis for which he is using cervical collar.
- History of motion sickness in childhood.
- Family history of migraine.
- No other relevant past family history.

On Examination
- Bilateral normal intact tympanic membrane.
- Rinne's test positive in both sides.
- Weber central.
- ABC normal.

CNS Examination
- No motor/sensory loss.
- No cranial nerve palsies.

- No abnormal cerebellar signs.
- Plantar flexor, knee jerk normal.
- Corneal reflex—normal in both sides.

Balance System

- Stepping test—slight rotation and deviated to right side more or less within normal limits.
- Gait—normal.
- Romberg's test—normal.
- Head shaking test—normal.
- No spontaneous, gaze and positional nystagmus.

Investigations

- Cardiac examinations—normal.
- Routine blood test—normal.
- Pure tone audiometry—within normal limit.
- ENG, ECG, VEMP—normal.
- MRI brain—normal.

Diagnosis

Migraine-related vertigo (MRV) as there is family history of migraine and a past history of motion sickness. Both these factors and the episodic vertigo with no aural symptoms suggest possibility of MRV.

Treatment

Since there is no definite clinical test to confirm it, a therapeutic trial with prophylactic antimigraine drugs such as flunarizine, amitryptyline and propranolol was instituted.

CASE 6: PERILYMPH FISTULA

A 45-year-old male patient met with a road traffic accident where he injured his head. CT head was normal. There was a transient loss of consciousness. There was no history of any ear bleeding. The patient was kept for observation overnight. He was discharged on the next day. He felt a little unstable but could walk. After 2 days, he started feeling unsteady while walking. There was mild rotator vertigo with no nausea or vomiting. The ear examination was essentially normal. Fistula sign was negative. Valsalva response was not recorded. He had tinnitus on the left side and high frequency sensorineural hearing loss (SNHL). Tympanogram showed a shallow A-type curve. High resolution computed tomography (HRCT) was repeated which showed no fracture lines or any damage to the otic capsule. He was initially treated on symptomatic treatment hoping that he will recover of his vestibular symptoms. However, his symptoms persisted. During this period, he had to travel by air. Though it was a short flight, his symptoms worsened and he had strong vertigo. He sought medical help and had to return by road. The sudden aggravation of symptoms raised suspicion of perilymph fistula. He was taken up for left exploratory tympanotomy. There was thin-fluid noted in the middle ear. It was sucked clear but re-accumulated within few minutes. On close observation, it was detected to be coming through fracture at the foot plate of stapes. The ossicles otherwise were intact. The fracture was not very obvious because of mucosal folds which were hiding the crack and the leak. The mucosa was swollen. It was divided and raised to either side. A small piece of tragal perichondrium was placed and mucosa replaced. It was not perfect cover by mucosa but enough to hold the graft position. A piece of gel foam under the crura through obturator foramen provided additional support to keep the tissues pressed against the foot plate at least for a few days. He was kept on bed rest with head elevated by 30° for 5 days. He was a Muslim by religion but was asked to avoid bending down during his prayers for a period of 3 weeks. His vestibular symptoms started improving the next day and became almost vertigo free in 2 weeks. He was not allowed to fly for 1 month. His hearing showed no improvement for the following 3 months. His tinnitus slowly reduced but did not go completely.

Point to learn in this case
- Post-head injury instability/vertigo can have varied presentations and causes including postconcussion syndrome. Some of them have confusion symptomatology. Often the investigations may not clinch the diagnosis.
- The aggravation of symptoms subsequent to sustained pressure variations are strong suggestion towards the diagnosis of perilymph fistula. Probably while testing fistula sign the pressure variations are not sustained long enough.
- Proactive approach towards exploratory tympanotomy should be the right way to manage these patients. Endomeatal tympanotomy is such a safe procedure that one can afford to have some negative explorations which should be acceptable.
- Hearing improvement and response to tinnitus may be poor. However, some patients do improve significantly, if intervened early.

CASE 7

A 42-year-old patient came to ENT-OPD with history of recurrent bouts of decreased hearing, tinnitus and vertigo. From history, it came to know that he has been suffering from recurrent bouts of vertigo for over 3 years and during this time, had consulted a number of general physicians, neurologists and general practitioners. He was told that there was an ear problem, but he was never referred to any ENT specialist. It was only now when his tinnitus became complicated did he come for an ENT check-up. On enquiry, he confessed to a feeling of aural fullness.

He had undergone different investigations and the only significant finding was a mild SNHL on audiometry.

He was advised a glycerol dehydration test and it came positive, confirming the diagnosis of Ménière's disease. He was advised proper medication like beta-histine/cinnarizine/prochlorperazine, mild diuretics and physiotherapy.

Comments

This patient was under treatment for long period, where every bout of vertigo of him was treated symptomatically with cinnarizine, beta-histine or prochlorperazine; however a diagnosis was never reached or attempted by the treating physicians. A simple test like audiometry was overlooked whereas MRI was done. This is a common scenario where the physicians fails to follow a protocol as far as both diagnosis and treatment are concerned.

CASE 8

A 55-year-old patient attended ENT-OPD with severe vertigo and hearing loss for only 1 day. Symptomatic treatment with intravenous prochlorperazine was given and an audiological evaluation was ordered. Pure tone audiometry revealed unilateral profound hearing loss. The treating doctor labeled it as Ménière's disease and put him on beta-histine and prochlorperazine. Eventually even when the vertigo subsided, the patient's hearing loss did not improve.

Comments

This is a patient of sudden sensorineural hearing loss who presented with acute vestibulocochlear pathology. The differentiating point here from Ménière's disease is the immediate development of profound hearing loss. Hearing could have possibly salvaged, if the patient was put on high dosage of steroid or intratympanic steroid.

CASE 9

A 50-year-old male executive reports with 3 episodes of sudden severe vertiginous sensations over a period of about a year, one of which lead to a fall. In that episode, the patient had fallen in the toilet and had sustained minor head injury for which he had to be hospitalized. Detailed history taking revealed that though he complained of vertigo, he did not actually have a typical rotating/spinning sensation. In the episode when he had fallen in the toilet, he had gone to the toilet at night, but after voiding, he suddenly fell down and all he could remember was that, he was lying flat on the floor of the toilet. Different clinical tests and investigations including MRI of the brain, MR angiography of the brain, ENG, CCG, carotid Doppler studies and EEG revealed nothing significant. On the two other occasions, he had a feeling of blankness in the head, profuse sweating, a sensation of nausea with spinning sensation in the head, a blurring of vision which gradually increased over a period of 1–2 minutes and finally a complete blackout. He did not have a fall but had lied down on the floor and after about 3–4 minutes, the symptoms subsided. All the attacks were aggravated while the person was standing. One of these episodes had taken place in his office while he was delivering a lecture. His friend reported to his wife that while lecturing he had suddenly complained that he was not feeling well and asked for a chair, but even before the chair could be brought, he lay down on the floor. He had become very pale in the face, with cold sweat in the forehead and his radial pulse had become very feeble and slow and later on was not palpable. After 15 minutes, when examined, nothing was abnormal except low blood pressure of 96/64 mm Hg. The patient complained of generalized weakness but no drowsiness at the time of examination.

General examination: It did not show any abnormality. Clinical neurotological tests were normal. Test for orthostatic hypotension, hyperventilation test and other dizziness revealed no abnormality.

Comments: This appears to be a case of syncope and not true balance disorder.

CASE 10

A 45-year-old male businessman, complained of instability, headache and vomiting for the last 3 months. He had an ataxic gait, ataxia in the left upper limb and papilledema.

Findings

- Caloric test findings showed a butterfly pattern of 1221.
- There is a left beating spontaneous nystagmus and gaze nystagmus to the left.
- The pendular eye tracking was grossly disorganized.
- The optokinetic nystagmus to the left was fairly normal while that to the right was grossly affected.

Comments

- Both the left beating caloric responses, e.g. L 440C and R 300C are hyperactive (directional preponderance to the left), while both the right beating caloric responses, e.g. R 440C and L 300C are hypoactive (inhibitory preponderance to the right).
- The directional preponderance suggests a disinhibitory lesion involving the temporal lobe of fibers projecting from it onto the left nystagmus generator in the brainstem.
- The suppression of the right beating caloric responses indicates a lesion in the brainstem involving the nystagmus generator on the right side responsible for producing right beating nystagmus.
- The patient was subsequently found to have a large brainstem tumor.

CHAPTER 12

Vertigo Clinic Evaluation Format

HISTORY

- Patient details
  - Name
  - Age
  - Sex
  - Address.
- Presenting complaint
  - Vertigo (surrounding/head-rotating),
  - Light headedness
  - Imbalance
  - Others.
- Duration of vertigo
  - Seconds
  - Hours
  - Days
  - Months
  - Years.
- Mode of onset
  - Sudden
  - Gradual.
- Associated symptoms
  - Nausea
  - Vomiting
  - Tinnitus

- Hearing loss
- Fullness in ear
- Blurring of vision
- Slurring of speech
- Headache
- Photophobia
- Others.
- Description of first attack.
- Frequency of each attack.
- Periods in between attacks.
  - Free of symptoms
  - Not free of symptoms.
- Warning signs before attack
  - Nil
  - Fullness in ear
  - Aura
  - Others.
- Aggravating factors
  - Nil
  - Coughing
  - Sneezing
  - Loud sounds
  - Specified food
  - Specific head position
  - Standing from sitting position
  - Turning in bed
  - Raising hands
  - Menstruation
  - Others.
- Relieving factors
  - Nil
  - Yes.
- Any URI/Fever before attack.

Vertigo Clinic Evaluation Format

- Headache
  - Yes
  - No.
- Cervical pain
  - Yes
  - No.
- Head injury/any trauma
  - Yes
  - No.
- Difficulty walking in the dark/streets/open spaces.
- Cardiovascular disorders
  - Yes (Hypertension/past history of MI/Palpitations/Chest pain/leg pain on walking or at rest/others)
  - No.
- Medical problems
  - No
  - Yes (Thyroid/diabetes mellitus/anemia/polycythemia/autoimmune/tuberculosis/smoking/alcohol/loss of weight/appetite/blood in stools/diarrhea/food intolerance/indigestion/bleeding disorders/microglobulinemia/others).
- Eye problems
  - No
  - Yes (Loss of vision/pain/discharge or tearing/glaucoma/diplopia/refractory errors/new glasses/others).
- Tullio phenomenon
  - Present
  - Absent.
- Ototoxic drugs/other medications
  - No
  - Yes.
- Acoustic trauma
  - No
  - Yes.

- Motion sickness
  - No
  - Yes.
- Psychiatric history
  - No
  - Yes (Insomnia/depression/conversion reaction/agoraphobia/others).
- Family history of giddiness/psych disease
  - No
  - Yes.
- History of unconsciousness
  - Yes
  - No.

If Patient Presents Like Near Faint

Sensation of impending faint (light headedness).

Mechanism: Diffuse cerebral ischemia (tunneling/dimming of vision, shortness of breath, air hunger, perioral numbness).

- *History of orthostatic hypotension:* Reduced blood volume, hypotensive drugs, autonomic dysfunction.
- *History of vasovagal attack:* Prolonged standing in hot sun, fear, severe pain, acute vertigo.
- *History of hyperventilation:* No/Yes (Anxiety, stress, panic attacks/associated symptoms-frequent sighing, air hunger/tightness in chest/perioral numbness/paresthesia of extremities).
- *History of reduced cardiac output:* No/Yes (Arrhythmia/valvular disease/heart failure).

Examinations

Systemic

- Pallor: Yes/No.

- *Blood pressure:* Lying/standing.
- *Bruits carotids:* No/Yes and Right/Left.

Ears

- *Tympanic membrane:* Right/Left.
- *Tuning fork test:* Right/Left, Webers-Right/Left, ABC-Right/Left.
- *Cranial nerves:*
  - Corneal reflex—right/left.
  - Eye movements—normal/abnormal.
  - Ptosis—no/Yes.
  - 7th, 9th, 10th, 11th, 12th cranial nerve examinations.
- *Neurological examination:*
  - *Deep tendon reflexes*—normal/abnormal.
  - *Babinsky*—normal/abnormal.
  - *Muscle strength*—normal/abnormal.
  - *Sensation on face*—normal/abnormal.
  - *Sensation on limbs*—normal/abnormal.
  - *Cerebellar functions*—finger to nose (with eyes open/eyes closed).
- *Examination of vestibulospinal system:*
  - Romberg's test (eye closed/eyes open).
  - Tandem standing test (eyes open/eyes closed).
  - Walking-tandem (eyes open/eyes closed).
  - Examination of gait.
- *Examination of vestibulo-ocular system:*
  - Opsoclonus—yes/no.
  - Ocular bobbing—yes/no.
  - Ocular flutter—yes/no.
  - Ocular myoclonus—yes/no.
  - Inspection of spontaneous nystagmus—no/yes (Horizontal—right/left, rotatory—clockwise/anticlockwise, vertical—up/down)—it is done with/without Frenzel lens and with/without optic fixation.

- Saccades—no/yes.
- Smooth pursuit—normal/abnormal.
- Headshaking nystagmus—no/yes.
- Positional testing—Dix-Hallpike maneuver.
- Valsalva-induced nystagmus—no/yes.
- Hyperventilation—dizziness (no/yes), nystagmus (no/yes).
- Tullio phenomenon—no/yes.
- Fistula test—no/yes.

Provisional diagnosis: We will get after history and examination.

INVESTIGATIONS

- Pure tone audiometry.
- Speech audiometry.
- Impedence audiometry.
- Acoustic reflex test.
- ENG.
- Blood tests—DC, TLC, Hb%, TSH, FBS, lipid profile, VDRL.
- Imaging—MRI/CT.
- Glycerol test (Right/Left).

Final diagnosis: We will get after all above steps.

MANAGEMENT

- Medications.
- Vestibular exercises.
- Surgery.

Points to Remember

PEARLS IN VERTIGO

- Vertigo is a symptom and not a disease, and it accounts for about 5% of all consultations with a general practitioner and 10–15% with an otorhinolaryngologist.
- *Vertigo* may be defined basically as a data mismatch in the sensory mechanism of the balance system consisting of visual, vestibular, acoustic, proprioceptive, CNS and peripheral nervous system.
- Dizziness is a nonspecific term which includes sense of imbalance (disequilibrium), blackout (presyncope), lightheadedness, floating sensation or vertigo.
- *Balance* is a complex interaction between the vestibular, ocular, proprioceptive and central nervous systems (CNS) to maintain head and body position in relation to the environment.
- Peripheral vestibular system is the vestibular apparatus which consists of the semicircular canals, utricle, saccule and the vestibular nerve.
- Central vestibular system includes vestibular nuclei and its central connections in the brainstem and cerebellum.
- Benign paroxysmal positional vertigo (BPPV) is the most frequent vestibular end organ disorder accounting for 20% of all dizziness cases.
- Dix-Hallpike test is the diagnostic test for BPPV.
- Medicines do not cure benign paroxysmal positional vertigo (BPPV) but are useful in controlling severe symptoms.
- *Benign paroxysmal positional vertigo (BPPV)* is often described self-limiting, because the symptoms subside or disappear even without treatment but, the recurrence rates are high.

- *Epley maneuver* is very beneficial in the management of BPPV.
- *Tullio's phenomenon* means feeling of vertigo on exposure to loud sounds. It may be seen Ménière's disease, perilymph fistula, fenestration and vestibulofibrosis.
- *Oscillopsia* is blurring of vision with head movement. It occurs with bilateral vestibular loss.
- Nystagmus is an involuntary movement of the eyes due to a disturbance vestibulo-ocular reflex (VOR). It can be due to either a peripheral or central vestibular disorder.
- Jerk nystagmus is the eye movement consists of a quick movement followed by a slow phase. The direction of nystagmus corresponds to the fast phase. Usually seen in peripheral vestibular disorders.
- Pendular nystagmus is the involuntary eye movement which has equal velocity in either direction. A sign of a central vestibular or congenital disorder.
- *Ménière's disease* is due raised endolymphatic pressure and clinically presents with episodic vertigo, low-pitched roaring tinnitus, fluctuating sensorineural hearing loss and sense of aural fullness.
- In early cases of Ménière's disease low frequencies sounds are affected more and the audiogram shows a rising curve. In long-standing cases, low and high frequencies are affected, audiogram becomes flat and then falling type.
- BPPV presents mostly in the fifth decade. It can follow an attack of vestibular neuronitis or head trauma or ear surgery. This is no gender bias.
- Acoustic neuroma is a slow growing tumor. There is concomitant vestibular adaptation and therefore severe vertigo does not occur.
- Vascular occlusion of labyrinthine artery is seen in the elderly with arteriosclerosis and those with hypercoagulation disease and cause irreversible hearing loss and episodic vertigo.

Points to Remember

- *Otolithic crisis of Tumarkin* or drop attacks are seen in early or late Ménière's disease. Patient feels as if pushed to the ground without any vertigo or loss of consciousness. It is presumed they are due to distortion of otolithic membrane of utricle or saccule when endolymphatic pressure rises.
- Positional nystagmus of peripheral origin occurs in a fixed direction, i.e. towards the undermost ear. Nystagmus of peripheral origin lasts only for a few seconds and is always less than one minute.
- On Dix-Hallpike testing, nystagmus of central origin appears immediately as soon as head is in critical position without a latent period.
- Cold water irrigation of ear canal causes nystagmus to opposite side and warm water to the same side (COWS).
- Ménière's disease is usually unilateral but other ear may be affected after a few years. Males are affected more than females.
- In Ménière's disease, during the initial vestibular excitation phase, the nystagmus will be ipsilateral but the vestibular depression phase, the nystagmus would beat towards the opposite side.
- Typically, a patient suffering from Ménière's disease would have a severe form of rotatory vertigo lasting a few hours with associated nausea and vomiting. Most of the time, there would not have been any precipitating factors. The attacks could occur anywhere and at any time of the day or night. Some patients might have a preceding sensation of fullness in the ear.
- In Ménière's disease, in between attacks the patient may not have any findings other than signs of sensorineural hearing loss (which again would be difficult to confirm clinically in the early stage of the disease).

- In vertigo patients, FTA-ABS should be done to rule out syphilitic cause.
- A vertical spontaneous nystagmus is always pathognomonic of a central vestibular lesion.
- Vestibular system generates the slow phase of nystagmus which is directed to the opposite side. The fast phase of the nystagmus is generated by the central nervous system.
- ENG does not measure or record torsional eye movements, which is characteristic of BPPV.
- The basis of the ENG testing is the corneo-retinal dipole, the cornea is the positive pole and the retina is the negative pole. ENG is not recommended for patients with less corneo-retinal potential difference (degenerative, diabetic or hypertensive retinopathies and retinitis pigmentosa) as the eye movement in these cases would be difficult to track by electrodes.
- A broad and wide-based gait with a tendency to fall, suggests the possibility of a cerebellar pathology.
- The most important point in the diagnosis of vertigo is an *unhurried and detailed history* (Professor Alan G Kerr).
- Hyperactive caloric response is seen in early Ménière's disease, central vestibular dysfunction. Decrease caloric response on the affected side is seen in unilateral vestibular dysfunction.
- The finger nose test and heel-knee test are tests to detect abnormalities of cerebellar function.
- During walking test, falling or deviating repeatedly in the same direction suggests an unilateral vestibular lesion on the side of fall.
- In *Unterburger's test*, the blind-folded patient is asked to extend his arms and step on the same spot alternately with each foot for 90 times in 1 minute. In peripheral vestibular lesions, the patient rotates/deviates to the side of the lesion; in central vestibular lesions, the sway is abnormally high.

- The vestibular rehabilitation exercises (also called Cawthrone-Cooksy exercises) are a must in the management of all patients of vestibular neuritis.
- *Cinnarizine* has a strong labyrinthine sedative effect and anti-vasoconstrictive effect. It reduces sludging phenomenon of blood in the narrow blood vessels and thereby reduces plasma viscosity which enhances microcirculation in the inner ear and in the brain.
- *Beta-histine* is the only non-sedating anti-vertigo drug available. It is used with caution in peptic ulcer and bronchial asthma patients.
- Use of cinnarizine in not contraindicated in peptic ulcer and bronchial asthma like beta-histine. Cinnarizine is very safe drug in geriatric patients.
- The slow phase of nystagmus is generated by the vestibular labyrinth (peripheral nervous system) and the fast phase of the nystagmus is generated by the central nervous system. The direction of the nystagmus is the direction of fast phase.
- Videonystagmography (VNG) can record rotator eye movement that is not possible by electronystagmography (ENG).
- The utricle is sensitive to horizontal displacement and the saccule is sensitive to vertical displacement.
- Falling or deviating repeatedly in the same direction suggests an unilateral vestibular lesion on the side of fall.
- The accuracy of timing, preciseness and perfect coordination of the muscular contraction of the extraocular and skeletal muscles is maintained by the cerebellum.
- Diuretics and low salt diet help in reducing the tension of endolymph in Ménière's disease.
- Equilibrium is maintained primarily by the vestibular part of labyrinth and is aided by visual and proprioceptive senses distributed all over the body. Final control of equilibrium is done by the cerebellum and cerebrum.

- Vertigo can occur from disorders of any of the three systems, vestibular, visual or somatosensory. Normally, the impulses reaching the brain from the three systems are equal and opposite. If any component on one side is inhibited or stimulated, the information reaching the higher center is mismatched leading to vertigo.
- *Lermoyez syndrome* has sensorineural hearing loss first followed by attacks of vertigo.
- Vestibular neuronitis is not accompanied by deafness but has severe vertigo of sudden onset.
- In acoustic neuroma, vertigo is not usually present or mild due to central adaptation.
- Any young adult presenting with unilateral sensorineural hearing loss and or tinnitus must be investigated with MRI/CT to rule out acoustic neuroma.
- *Key points of vestibular neuronitis:*
  - Vestibular neuronitis has sudden onset.
  - Only vestibular system is affected.
  - There is severe rotatory vertigo at onset.
  - There is gradual recovery with time.
- *Key points of benign paroxysmal positional vertigo:*
  - It is the most common vestibular disorder.
  - Rotatory vertigo is of short duration.
  - It is normally easy to provoke.
  - It is usually self-limiting.
  - It may be treated with rotator maneuver.
- History taking remains the main weapon for diagnosis of a patient with balance disorder.
- Cardiovascular causes of dizziness are vasovagal syncope, orthostatic hypotension, embolic disease and cardiac dysrhythmias.
- Endocrine causes of dizziness are hypoglycemia, adrenal failure and pheochromocytoma.

- *Presbystasis* is the progressive loss of balance function accompanies the normal aging process.
- *Hennebert's sign:* Nystagmus induced by pressure insufflations against an intact tympanic membrane. It is a false positive fistula sign. First described in patient with congenital syphilis due to a hypermobile stapes foot plate. Also noted in Ménière's disease, where it causes stapes footplate movement, the undersurface of which is adhered to the distended saccule.
- Vestibular neuritis or neuronitis is a viral infection of the vestibular nerve or vestibular (Scarpa's) ganglion. It is most commonly thought to be due to Herpes simplex type I viral infection.
- Electronystagmography (ENG) is not recommended for patients with less corneo-retinal potential difference (degenerative, diabetic or hypertensive retinopathies and retinitis pigmentosa) as the eye movements in these cases would be difficult to track by electrodes. ENG does not measure or record torsional eye movements, which is characteristic of benign paroxysmal positional vertigo.
- Treatment of acute attack of Ménière's disease is primarily aimed at control of vertigo and vomiting. Prochlorperazine and ondansetron are commonly preferred medications for control of vomiting. Vertigo control requires the use of vestibular suppressants like connarizine or prochlorperazine for 3–5 days.
- Prolonged use of vestibular suppressants is not advisable as this may hamper vestibular compensation and thus delay recovery.
- People with Ménière's disease are advised to avoid high salt containing food like papad, pickles, etc. Consumption of alcohol and chocolates, and nicotine use is discouraged.
- In Ménière's disease, diuretic whenever prescribed should preferably be the potassium sparing variety triamterene.

Loop diuretics are unsafe in our country for risk of hyponatremia and hypokalemia. Many prefer to use acetazolamide for short periods of time.
- At least 2 definitive episodes of vertigo of at least 20 minutes duration must have occurred to make the diagnosis of Ménière's disease. Duration is usually several hours long.
- In Ménière's disease, pure tone audiometry shows a low frequency or mixed low and high frequency loss may develop. Typically, lower frequencies are affected more often than higher frequencies because of preferential sensitivity of the apex to hydrops.
- Dysdiadochokinesia is the inability to perform rapidly alternating motor movements, a sign of cerebellar disease.
- The characteristic of the nystagmus that is diagnostic of BPPV is that it is *latent* (starts after 10–15 seconds), *short lasting* (lasts for about 15–20 seconds), *rotatory* (is mixed vertical-torsional), *geotropic* (the direction of rotation of eyeballs is towards the floor with the affected ear down), *fatigable* (tends to fade away on repeating the test multiple times) and *reversible* (upon rapidly bringing the patient to sitting position, many times a milder rotator nystagmus is elicited opposite to that in supine head-hanging position).
- Before doing Dix-Hallpike test, it is important to rule out, if the patient is having any significant complaint of cervical spine or any history of coronary artery disease, in which cases the test is modified.
- *Wallenberg's syndrome (Lateral medullary syndrome or PICA syndrome; most common brainstem stroke):* The patient presents with vertigo, ataxia, dysarthria and unilateral Horner's syndrome (ptosis, meiosis and anhidrosis). *Anterior cerebellar artery (AICA) strokes:* The patient presents with vertigo and unilateral deafness. Isolated pontine infarcts may present with vertigo alone and may mimic vestibular neuritis.

- In Ménière's disease, medical therapy has been the mainstay of treatment and surgical option is reserved for the cases that did not improve with conservative therapy. Medical therapy includes low-salt diet and diuretics.
- In Ménière's disease, smoking and excessive stress are discouraged as these are precipitating factors. The patient is also instructed to avoid canned foods, cheese and pickles.
- In Ménière's disease, surgery is considered in cases with rapid progression of the disease and in those who did not respond to conservative therapy. Surgical options include hearing preservation surgeries such as endolymphatic sac decompression and retrolabyrinthine or middle fossa selective vestibular nerve section. Hearing destructive surgeries can be performed in patients with severe to profound hearing loss and include labyrinthecomy and translabyrinthine VIII nerve section.
- Endolymphatic sac surgery is widely used as the primary surgical procedure at various centers around the world and success for the surgery has been reported to be between 60% and 80% by various authors.
- Migraine is the most common cause of headache in the world. Prevalence studies have shown that 14–22% of women and 5–8% of men suffer from migraine.
- Blood tests can be advised when the clinical diagnosis is Ménière's disease to distinguish between syphilis—a condition in which ear symptoms resemble Ménière's. However, this does not mean that every Ménière's patient should be suspected for syphilis.
- A unilateral or asymmetrical sensorineural hearing loss is an indication for imaging to exclude a tumor of the VII cranial nerve. Gadolinium MRI is the imaging of choice.
- The vestibular apparatus consists of the semicircular canals, utricle, saccule and the vestibular nerve. The otolithic organs

consist of the utricle, which is adjacent to the semicircular canals and the saccule which is close to the cochlea.
- The sensory neuroepithelium is called the crista in the semicircular canals and the macula in the otolithic organs.
- The crista within the ampula consists of hair cells embedded in a gelatinous substance called the *cupula*. The semicircular canals determine rotational velocity in three dimensions.
- The macula within the utricle and saccule contain hair cells coupled to calcium carbonate crystals called *otoconia* or *otoliths*. They sense gravity and linear accelerations.
- A defect in the vestibule-ocular reflex results in nystagmus. Nystagmus consists of involuntary eye movements with a fast and a slow component. The direction of the nystagmus follows the direction of the fast phase.
- *Pendular nystagmus:* Beats of similar velocity each direction (central cause). *Jerk nystagmus:* Quick and slow phase (Peripheral vestibular or central cause).
- In a peripheral vestibular lesion, where there is hyperactivity on the side of the lesion the nystagmus beats towards the side of the lesion (the stronger ear).
- In Ménière's disease, there is an initial irritative phase where the nystagmus beats towards the side of the lesion. The direction of the nystagmus changes to beat away from the side of the affected ear later in the paretic phase, where there is hypoactivity of the affected side.
- *Horizontal nystagmus of peripheral origin (Labyrinth or VIII nerve) obeys Alexander's law which states the nystagmus:* It always in one direction, irrespective of the direction of gaze and Intensity of the nystagmus is greatest when looking in the direction of the fast phase.
- Prochlorperazine is the most effective drug for controlling acute vertigo. This drug is best used for a very short course to relieve acute symptoms, but should preferably be discontinued

as soon as the acute symptoms subside such that the vestibular compensation is not inhibited.
- Beta-histine is used with caution in peptic ulcer and bronchial asthma patients.
- A nystagmus generated by a central vestibular pathology often (but not always) increases in intensity when the eyes are open (i.e. optic fixation) and decreases when the eyes are closed. If intensity of nystagmus decreases on optic fixation, it is usually a peripheral vestibular lesion but a central lesion is also possible.
- A broad and wide-based gait with a tendency to fall, suggests the possibility of a cerebellar pathology. Falling or deviating repeatedly in the same direction suggests an unilateral vestibular lesion on the side of fall.
- Onset of vertigo is sudden in peripheral vestibular lesion whereas gradual onset in central pathology.
- If the positional nystagmus does not have a latent period, then its direction changing, not accompanied by an appreciable sensation of vertigo and is not fatiguable, then this is expected to be of central origin.

Bibliography

1. Biswas A. An Introduction to Neurotology.
2. Baloh RW, Fife TD, Furman JM, et al. The approach to the patient with dizziness.
3. Baloh RW. Episodic vertigo: Central nervous system causes. Current Opinion in Neurology. 2002;15:17-21.
4. Baloh RW. Vertigo. Lancet. 1998;352;1841-6.
5. Bojrab DI, et al. Peripheral vestibular disorders. Jackler and Brackmann Neurotology. 2004;36;629-50.
6. Brandt T, Daroff RB. Physical therapy for benign paroxysmal positional vertigo. Arch Otolaryngol. 1980;106-484-5.
7. Brandt T, Dieterich M, Strupp M. Vertigo and Dizziness. Springerlink. 2005.
8. Brandt T, et al. Vertigo and Dizziness: common complaints. Springer 2005.
9. Clinical Neurotology. Diagnosing and managing disorders of hearing, balance and the facial nerve. In: Lustig LR, Niparko JK, Minor LB, Zee DS (Eds). New York: Martin Duntiz, 2003.
10. Mathur NN. Common Vestibulocochlear Disorders.
11. Cutrer FM, Baloh RW. Migraine associated dizziness. Headache. 1992;32:300-4.
12. Desmond Alan. Vestibular Function: Evaluation and Treatment. Thieme Medical Publishers Inc, New York, 2004.
13. Garia Vaz F. Vertigo. Nine Clinical Cases. 2000. pp. 53-68.
14. Guilemany JM, et al. Clinical and epidemiological study of vertigo at an outpatient clinic. Acta Otorhinolaryngol Ital. 2004;124(1):49-52.
15. Hain TC, Yacovino D. Pharmacologic treatment of persons with dizziness. Neurologic Clin. 2005;23:831-53.

16. Hamid M, Sismanis A. Medical Otology and Neurotology: a Clinical Guide to Auditory and Vestibular Disorders. New York: Thieme; 2006.
17. Kerr AG. Teaching labyrinthine vertigo to medical students. Estratto do Minerva Otorhinolaryngologica. 1975;25:147-53.
18. Lalwani AK. Current diagnosis and treatment. Otolaryngology Head and Neck Surgery, 2nd ed.
19. Neuhauser HK. Epidemiology of vertigo. Curr Opin Neurol. 2007;20:40-46.
20. Paine M. Dealing with Dizziness. Australian Prescriber. 2005;28:94-7.
21. Devesahayam PR, Narayanan P. Vertigo: Clinical Practice and Examination.
22. Post RE, Dickerson LE. Dizziness: a diagnostic approach. Am Fam Physcian. 2010;82:361-8.
23. Post RE, Dickerson LM. Dizziness: a diagnostic approach. Am Fam Physcian. 2010;82(4):361-9.
24. Ruckenstein MJ, Staab J. Chronic subjective dizziness. Otolaryngol Clin N Am. 2009;42:71-77.
25. Scott Brown's Otolaryngology, Head and Neck Surgery, 7th edn, vol 3: p.3798.
26. Swartz R, Longwell P. Treatment of Vertigo. Am Fam Physcian. 2005;71:1115-22.
27. Weber PC. Vertigo and Disequilibrium: A Practical Guide to Diagnosis and Management. New York: Thieme; 2007.
28. White J. Benign paroxysmal positional vertigo: how to diagnose and quickly treat it. Cleve Clin J Med. 2004;71:722-8.

Index

Page numbers followed by *f* refer to figure and *t* refer to table

A

ABC test 40
Agoraphobia 4, 12
Alexander's law 41
American Institute of Health Statistics 4
Aminoglycosides 30
Amitriptyline 73
Ampullary nerve section 83
Anemia 21
Anxiety neurosis 4
Arrhythmias 12
Arthritis 30
Asthma, bronchial 74
Ataxia 10
    cerebellar 31
Atrophy, cerebellar 33
Audio-evoked response 60
Audiological test 55
Autophony 102

B

Babinski's test 40
Barbiturates 30
Bechterew's nucleus 7
Blood pressure 30, 37, 117, 135
Blood sugar, fasting 55, 118
Blood urea 55, 118
Brain tumor 30
Brainstem
    concussion 27
    hemorrhage 12
    infarct 33
    ischemia 106
    tumors of 13, 19
Brandt-Daroff exercise 78, 78*f*

C

Calcium channel blocker 72-75
Caloric test 21, 59, 60*f*, 118
Cardiovascular disease 116
Cardiovascular system 10
Cawthrone-Cooksey exercises 79, 86, 141
Central nervous system 2, 10, 21, 137
Cerebellar artery syndrome, posterior-inferior 13, 18
Cerebellar function tests 40, 135
Cerebellar test 53, 118
Cerebrovascular disease 22
Cervical pain 133
Chiari malformations 44
Claussen butterfly chart 58*f*
Cogan's syndrome 104
Corneal reflex 43, 135
Cranial nerve 117, 135
Craniocorpography 57, 58

D

Diabetes mellitus 12
Diplopia 12, 32, 33
Dix-Hallpike test 47, 49f, 118, 120, 137
    steps of 48f
Dizziness 23, 25, 113
    common causes of 12
    episodic 110
Drop attacks 32
Dysarthria 32, 33
Dysdiadochokinesia 53, 118
Dysesthesia 32
Dysmetria 32
Dysphagia 32, 33

E

Electrocardiogram 118
Electrocochleography 60, 118
Electronystagmography 57, 120, 141, 143
Endolymphatic sac surgery 82
Enzymes 55, 118
Epilepsy 13
    temporal lobe 20
Epley maneuver 66, 76, 138
    steps in 77f
Epstein-Barr virus 12
Erythrocyte sedimentation rate 55, 104
Eustachian tube 102
Exercises
    adaptation 86
    compensation 86
    convergence 86, 88f
    eye 86
    head and neck 88
    vestibular 136
Eye cover test 53

F

Fistula
    labyrinthine 66
    perilymph 11, 12, 15, 26, 27, 36, 65, 100, 126
    sign
        false negative 44
        false positive 44
    test 43, 102, 118, 136
Flunarizine 73
Fluorescent treponemal antibody 55, 68
Fluoxetine 73
Frenzel's glass 41, 41f
Friedreich's ataxia 12

G

Gait 118
    ataxia 31
    examination of 135
Gaze test 120
Glycerol test 56, 121, 136

H

Halmagyi test 51
Head impulse 51
Head injury 15, 30, 133
Head movements 81

Head shake test 46, 47f, 117
Headache 132, 133
Heart disease 30
Hemorrhage 105
  cerebellar 33
Hennebert's sign 101, 102, 143
Horner's syndrome 105
Human immune deficiency virus 12
Hydrochlorothiazide 73
Hypertension 30
Hyperventilation 31, 134, 136
  syndrome 12
Hypoglycemia 21, 30, 114
Hypotension 12
  orthostatic 21, 50, 134
  postural 31, 37, 117

I

Infarction, cerebellar 22, 105
Inflammatory diseases 64
Inner ear disease, autoimmune 33
Ischemia
  cerebral 107
  labyrinthine 33
  vertebrobasilar 33

L

Labyrinth
  bilateral complete depression of 18
  intermittent failure of 65
  irritation of 65
  unilateral complete depression of 17
  unilateral incomplete depression of 17
Labyrinthectomy 82
Labyrinthine artery, vascular occlusion of 138
Labyrinthitis 11-13, 15, 26, 30, 33, 36, 102
  autoimmune 104
  infective 71
  syphilitic 12, 68
Lermoyez syndrome 142

M

Ménière's disease 11-13, 16, 17, 26, 29, 33, 34, 36, 56, 63, 65, 67, 68, 70, 73, 82, 83, 96, 97, 111, 112, 120, 123, 138, 139, 140, 141, 143
Ménière's triad 96t
Metabolic disease 116
Metoclopramide 73
Metronidazole 15
Migraine 12, 30, 33, 34, 116
  basilar artery 19
Motion sickness 22, 36, 107, 134
Muscle strength 135
Multiple sclerosis 12, 13, 19, 26, 33, 71, 106
Myoclonus, ocular 42, 135

N

Nalidixic acid 15
Nausea 10
Neuritis, vestibular 12, 33, 70, 73, 143
Neuroma, acoustic 11, 13, 16, 36, 102, 103f, 138

Neuronitis, vestibular 11, 13, 14, 17, 26, 30, 36, 99, 119, 142, 143
Nystagmus 10, 138
    central and peripheral 41, 42, 42*t*
    gaze-evoked 117
    head shaking 136
    jerk 138, 146
    pendular 138, 146
    peripheral 42
    pure vertical 40
    spontaneous 40, 42*f*, 117
    Valsalva induced 136

O

Ocular dysfunction, vestibular 12
Oculomotor tests 52, 117
Opsoclonus 42, 135
Optokinetic test 59
Oscillopsia test 50
Otolith-ocular reflexes 118
Otorrhea 30
Otoscopy 117
Ototoxicity 23, 36

P

Pallor 37, 117
Panic disorders 12
Peptic ulcer 74
Pheochromocytoma 74
Photophobia 132
Pinna and external auditory canal, examination of 38
Plantar flexor 122
Polyarteritis nodosa 104
Positron emission tomography 55
Postconcussion syndrome 27
Prednisolone 73
Presbystasis 143
Presyncope 12
Promethazine 73
Psychiatric disorders 12
Ptosis 135
Pure tone audiometry 55, 118, 136

R

Red blood cells 74
Rehabilitation exercises, vestibular 85
Rehabilitation therapy, vestibular 79
Rinne's test 39, 117
Romberg test 45, 118, 135
Rotation test 46
Rotation, sensation of 3

S

Saccades 52, 136
Scarpa's ganglion 7
Schwalbe's nucleus 7
Selective serotonin reuptake inhibitor 73
Semont maneuver 79
Sensorineural hearing loss 126
Single photon emission computerized tomography 55
Speech audiometry 136
Spinal nucleus 7

Spondylosis, cervical 30
Spondylotic myelopathy, cervical 31
Steroids, intratympanic 82
Stimulation
    caloric 17
    labyrinthine 16
Stroke
    cerebellar 26
    inferior cerebellar 12
Suppurative otitis media, chronic 65
Syphilis 11, 16
Systemic lupus erythematosus 104

T

Tandem standing test 135
Tendon reflexes, deep 40, 122, 135
Thyroid dysfunction 12
Thyroid function test 55, 118
Transient Ischemic attack 12, 106
Trauma 64
    acoustic 133
    labyrinthine 13, 36
Traumatic head injury 12
Tricyclic antidepressants 73, 75
Trifluopromazine 73
Tullio's phenomenon 100-102, 133, 136, 138
Tumor, cerebellar 33
Tuning fork test 39, 122, 135

U

Unconsciousness 134
Unsteadiness, sensation of 3

Unterburger's test 45, 46f, 120, 140
Utricular dysfunction 118

V

Valsalva maneuver 44
Vascular diseases 64
Vascular insufficiency 107
Vasovagal attack 31, 134
Venereal disease research laboratory 55, 118
Vertebrobasilar insufficiency 13, 18, 66, 67, 71, 106
Vertebrobasilar transient ischemic attack 34
Vertigo 3, 10, 35, 37, 55, 62, 74, 109, 111
    alternobaric 12, 66, 67
    benign paroxysmal 11-14, 17, 36, 63, 99, 122, 137, 142
    benign positional 11-14, 17, 26, 36, 63, 66, 99, 122, 137, 142
    causes of 11, 20
    central causes of 32, 33, 104
    cervical 12, 13, 20
    clinic evaluation format 131
    diagnosis 35
    epileptic 71
    labyrinthine 16
    migrainous 26, 105
    non-recurrent 30
    ocular 20
    onset of 29
    otologic 111
    ototoxic 13
    peripheral 21, 34t

physiological 5, 22
post-traumatic 25
psychogenic 20
rotatory 66
treatment of 62
true 112
with deafness 13, 36
without deafness 13, 36
Vestibular disorders
central 18
peripheral 12, 13
Vestibular evoked myogenic potentials 59, 118
Vestibular origin, peripheral 11
Vestibular system, disorders of 11
Vestibule-spinal reflex, assessment of 57
Vestibule-spinal system, examination of 135
Vestibulocerebellar tracts 10
Vestibulo-ocular reflex 9, 10, 51, 138
assessment of 57
Vestibulo-ocular system, examination of 135
Vestibulopathy, bilateral 12, 103
Vestibulospinal tract 10, 118
Vestibulotoxic drugs 11, 15
Video head impulse test 118
Videonystagmography 57, 141
Vision, blurring of 132
Vomiting 10

W

Walking test 45
Wallenberg's syndrome 18, 105, 144
Weber's test 39, 117
Whiplash injury 27

EU GSPR Authorised Reprsentative
Logos Europe, 9 rue Nicolas Poussin
1700, La Rochelle, France
Phone: +33 (0) 6 67 93 73 78
E-mail: contact@logoseurope.eu

www.ingramcontent.com/pod-product-compliance
Ingram Content Group UK Ltd.
Pitfield, Milton Keynes, MK11 3LW, UK
UKHW022000190326
4862IPUK00003B/25